Health, Behaviour and Society: Clinical Medicine in Context

Titles in the Series

Professional Practice for Foundation Doctors   ISBN 9780857252845
Succeeding in Your Medical Degree   ISBN 9780857253972
Law and Ethics in Medical Practice   ISBN 9780857250988
Critical Thinking and Research for Medical Students   ISBN 9780857256010

To order, please contact our distributor: BEBC Distribution, Albion Close, Parkstone, Poole, BH12 3LL. Telephone: 0845 230 9000, email: learningmatters@bebc.co.uk.
You can also find more information on each of these titles and our other learning resources at www.learningmatters.co.uk

Health, Behaviour and Society: Clinical Medicine in Context

Editors: Jennifer Cleland and Philip Cotton

Series Editors:
Judy McKimm and Kirsty Forrest

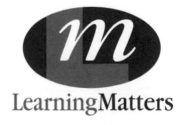

© 2011 Chapter 1, Jennifer Cleland, Shirley Laird and Blair Smith; Chapter 2, Jennifer Cleland and Jane Smith; Chapter 3, Jane Smith and Jennifer Cleland; Chapter 4, Maureen A. Porter and Edwin van Teijlingen; Chapter 5, Karen Foster, Cairns Smith and Edwin van Teijlingen; Chapter 6, Cairns Smith and Finlay Dick; Chapter 7, Philip Cotton and Lindsey Pope; Chapter 8, Philip Cotton, Jim McKillop and Jennifer Cleland; Chapter 9, Lindsey Pope and Philip Cotton.

The rights of Jennifer Cleland, Shirley Laird, Blair Smith, Jane Smith, Maureen A. Porter, Edwin van Teijlingen, Karen Foster, Cairns Smith, Finlay Dick, Philip Cotton, Lindsey Pope and Jim McKillop to be identified as Authors of this Work (as listed above) have been asserted by them in accordance with the Copyright, Designs and Patents Act 1988.

British Library Cataloguing in Publication Data
A CIP record for this book is available from the British Library.

ISBN 9780857254610

This book is also available in the following ebook formats:
AER ISBN 9780857254634
EPUB ISBN 9780857254627
Kindle ISBN 9780857254641

Cover and text design by Code 5 Design Associates
Project management by Swales & Willis Ltd, Exeter, Devon
Typeset by Swales & Willis Ltd, Exeter, Devon
Printed and bound in Great Britain by Short Run Press Ltd, Exeter, Devon

Learning Matters Ltd
20 Cathedral Yard
Exeter EX1 1HB
Tel: 01392 215560
info@learningmatters.co.uk
www.learningmatters.co.uk

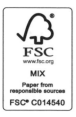

FSC
www.fsc.org
MIX
Paper from
responsible sources
FSC® C014540

For Alexandra, Ollie and Kate

Contents

Foreword from the Series Editors   viii
Author Biographies   x

Introduction   1
Jennifer Cleland and Philip Cotton

Part 1   The Doctor as a Scholar and a Scientist   5

Chapter 1   An Introduction to Health and Illness in Society   7
             Jennifer Cleland, Shirley Laird and Blair Smith

Chapter 2   Using Psychology to Help Your Medical Practice   25
             Jennifer Cleland and Jane Smith

Chapter 3   The Interaction of Psychological Factors with Illness,
             Disease and Treatment   44
             Jane Smith and Jennifer Cleland

Chapter 4   The Sociology of Health and Illness   61
             Maureen A. Porter and Edwin van Teijlingen

Chapter 5   Populations, Health and Disease   79
             Karen Foster, Cairns Smith and Edwin van Teijlingen

Chapter 6   Promoting and Improving Health at a Population Level   99
             Cairns Smith and Finlay Dick

Part 2   Applying Knowledge to Clinical Practice   119

Chapter 7   Scientific Method and Critical Appraisal   121
             Philip Cotton and Lindsey Pope

Chapter 8   Activity Limitation and Disability   141
             Philip Cotton, Jim McKillop and Jennifer Cleland

Chapter 9   Pulling It All Together   159
             Lindsey Pope and Philip Cotton

             References   177
             Index   184

Foreword from the Series Editors

The Learning Matters Medical Education Series

Medical education is currently experiencing yet another a period of change typified in the UK with the introduction of the revised *Tomorrow's Doctors* (General Medical Council, 2009) and ongoing work on establishing core curricula for many subject areas. This new series of textbooks has been developed as a direct response to these changes and the impact on undergraduate medical education.

Research indicates that effective medical practitioners combine excellent, up-to-date clinical and scientific knowledge with practical skills and the ability to work with patients, families and other professionals with empathy and understanding, they know when to lead and when to follow and they work collaboratively and professionally to improve health outcomes for individuals and communities. The General Medical Council has defined a series of learning outcomes set out under three headings:

- Doctor as Practitioner
- Doctor as Scholar and Scientist
- Doctor as Professional

The books in this series do not cover practical clinical procedures or knowledge about diseases and conditions, but instead cover the range of non-technical professional skills (plus underpinning knowledge) that students and doctors need to know in order to become effective, safe and competent practitioners.

Aimed specifically at medical students (but also of use for junior doctors, teachers and clinicians), each book relates to specific outcomes of *Tomorrow's Doctors*, providing both knowledge and help to improve the skills necessary to be successful at the non-clinical aspects of training as a doctor. One of the aims of the series is to set medical practice within the wider social, policy and organisational agendas to help produce future doctors who are socially aware and willing and prepared to engage in broader issues relating to healthcare delivery.

Individual books in the series outline the key theoretical approaches and policy agendas relevant to that subject, and go further by demonstrating through case studies and scenarios how these theories can be used in work settings to achieve best practice. Plenty of activities and self-assessment tools throughout the book will help the reader to hone their critical thinking and reflection skills.

Chapters in each of the books follow a standard format. At the beginning a box highlights links to relevant competencies and outcomes from *Tomorrow's Doctors* and other medical curricula if appropriate. This sets the scene and enables the reader to see exactly what will be covered. This is extended by a chapter overview which sets out the key topics and what the student should expect to have learnt by the end of the chapter.

There is at least one case study in each chapter which considers how theory can be used in practice from different perspectives. Activities are included which include practical tasks with learning points, critical thinking research tasks and reflective practice/thinking points. Activities can be carried out by the reader or with others and are designed to raise awareness, consolidate understanding of theories and ideas and enable the student to improve their practice by using models, approaches and ideas. Each activity is followed by a brief discussion on issues raised. At the end of each chapter a chapter summary provides an aide-memoire of what has been covered.

All chapters are evidence based in that they set out the theories or evidence that underpins practice. In most chapters, one or more 'What's the evidence?' boxes provide further information about a particular piece of research or a policy agenda through books, articles, websites or policy papers. A list of additional readings is set out under the 'Going further' section, with all references collated at the end of the book.

The series is edited by Professor Judy McKimm and Dr Kirsty Forrest, both of whom are experienced medical educators and writers. Book and chapter authors are drawn from a wide pool of practising clinicians and educators from the UK and internationally.

Author Biographies

Jennifer Cleland

Jennifer Cleland is a Clinical Senior Lecturer in medical education and primary care at the University of Aberdeen and an Honorary Clinical Psychologist in Liaison Psychiatry to NHS Grampian. She runs the Clinical Communication vertical theme and oversees Years 1–3 of Community Medicine. Her main research interests are in developing and evaluating educational interventions at all stages of medical training and practice.

Philip Cotton

Philip Cotton is a General Practitioner with a special interest in supporting victims of torture. He is Deputy Head of the Medical School and Associate Dean for Student Welfare (Medicine) at Glasgow University. He has an active involvement in international medical education and his main research interest is medical education.

Finlay Dick

Finlay Dick is a Senior Lecturer in Occupational Medicine at the University of Aberdeen and an Honorary Consultant Occupational Physician to NHS Grampian. His main research interests are occupational and environmental risk factors, and gene-environment interactions in Parkinson's Disease.

Karen Foster

Karen Foster has worked both as a General Practitioner and as a Consultant in Public Health Medicine. She is currently the Teaching Co-ordinator for General Practice and Community Medical Education at the University of Aberdeen.

Shirley Laird

Shirley Laird is a GP locum in Aberdeen, Scotland and a Clinical Senior Lecturer in the Centre of Academic Primary Care at the University of Aberdeen. She has responsibility for the academic co-ordination and development of the Community Course, which encompasses the specialties of General Practice, Child Health, Psychiatry, Medicine for the Elderly, Occupational/Environmental Health and Public Health in the first three years of the undergraduate curriculum.

Jim McKillop

Jim McKillop is Muirhead Professor of Medicine at the University of Glasgow and Chair of the GMC Undergraduate Board. His professional activities have focussed on internal medicine, nuclear medicine and medical education. He has a personal interest in disability based on his own polio-related disability. He teaches undergraduate medical students on this topic, has chaired a Scottish Government Working Group on Post-Polio Services and chairs the Expert Panel of the British Polio Fellowship.

Lindsey Pope

Lindsey Pope is a Clinical University Teacher at the University of Glasgow. She runs the Clinical Practice in the Community and Communication Skills Courses. Clinically, she is a GP in Port Glasgow in a practice which trains both medical students and GP specialist trainees.

Maureen A. Porter

Maureen Porter is a medical sociologist who has spent many years researching aspects of women's reproductive health. She is now a Teaching Fellow at Aberdeen University's Division of Medical and Dental Education co-ordinating courses in the sociology of health and illness and qualitative research methods and supervising postgraduate students.

Blair Smith

Blair Smith is a general practitioner in Peterhead, Scotland, and Professor of General Practice, University of Aberdeen. He is Head of General Practice and Community Medical Education at the University of Aberdeen, where he led the development of the Community Course, integrating clinical, behavioural and social sciences for undergraduate medical students.

Cairns Smith

Cairns Smith is Professor of Public Health at the University of Aberdeen. He is also a Consultant in Public Health with NHS Grampian with responsibilities for training, health promotion and health protection. His main research interests are in the epidemiology and control of both communicable and non-communicable chronic disease.

Jane Smith

Jane Smith is a Lecturer in Health Psychology at the Norwich Medical School in the Faculty of Medicine & Health Sciences at the University of East Anglia (UEA). Her research and teaching interests primarily cover psychosocial aspects of chronic disease prevention and management.

Edwin van Teijlingen

Edwin van Teijlingen is a medical sociologist with an interest in public health. He is Professor of Reproductive Health Research at Bournemouth University and has taught medical students at universities in the UK and in Nepal.

Introduction

Jennifer Cleland and Philip Cotton

In *Good Medical Practice* the GMC (2006, p6) states:

> *Good doctors make the care of their patients their first concern: they are competent,*
> *keep their knowledge and skills up to date, establish and maintain good relationships*
> *with patients and colleagues, are honest and trustworthy, and act with integrity.*

Care of a person is more than treating a particular symptom or disease: patients
are individuals but they are often part of a family or small group, of a community,
and live within a particular environment and context. All these factors can affect
in many different ways how people experience and manage health and illness. This
book introduces the learner to patients, some of whom will have a physical illness but
many of whom, particularly those presenting in the community, are physically 'normal' with problems rooted in psychological or environmental causes. It illustrates
that medicine involves more than just getting rid of physical illness; rather it includes
improving or maximising the potential of other aspects of the patient's life. The content crosses traditional medical specialty boundaries: perspectives from all the
'community-based' disciplines are introduced and integrated. Why have we taken a
community perspective? It is estimated that between 90 and 95 per cent of people are
managed completely in general practice, and in one year 70 per cent of people will
see their GP and over 90 per cent of under-fives will be brought to community-based
healthcare settings including general practice.

This book helps to address *Tomorrow's Doctors*: outcomes and standards for undergraduate medical education (GMC, 2009) competencies relating to core attributes of
the Doctor as Scientist and Scholar. Throughout the book, content is mapped against
the key areas of psychology, sociology and population health set out in this theme.
Reflecting *Tomorrow's Doctors* (2009), patient safety, service improvement, ethical and
best clinical practice are key aspects of this book, and differentiate this book from others that focus either on clinical aspects or on more detailed generic skills.

This book introduces key concepts in the areas of psychological, sociological and
population influences on health, starting with normality and moving to illness and
disease. Key influences on health and healthcare are discussed from the individual to
the population so readers place the patient who presents in clinic to the wider context of healthcare.

The book will cover the context of care and the systems of care in the UK, and
compare these to international healthcare models – political, social and economic
– to illustrate global differences in health and healthcare.

The book also covers the scientific basis of medicine and provides guidance
on research skills and critical appraisal. These topics are now being emphasised at

undergraduate levels and in the Foundation curriculum. Furthermore, several key aspects of developing as a professional, including reflective practice, are covered.

Who should read this book?

This book is designed to support medical students during their undergraduate studies and in preparation and application for Foundation Training posts. It may be particularly relevant early in a student's learning but will provide guidance to help medical students in all years make sense of *Tomorrow's Doctors* (2009), and assess how *Tomorrow's Doctors* (2009) applies to them. It is also useful for international medical students and doctors wishing to apply to transfer into undergraduate courses, train or work in the UK. It is also a useful resource for programme developers in UK and international medical schools.

Book structure

The book is structured in two parts, each of which has a number of chapters. The topics covered are those arising from *Tomorrow's Doctors* (2009), Outcomes 9–12:

- *The doctor as a scholar and a scientist*:
  - Apply psychological principles, method and knowledge to medical practice
  - Apply social science principles, method and knowledge to medical practice
  - Apply to medical practice the principles, method and knowledge of population health and the improvement of health and healthcare
  - Apply scientific method and approaches to medical research
- *Applying knowledge to clinical practice*

Part 1: The Doctor as a Scholar and a Scientist

Chapters 1–6 introduce a broad approach to patient care and medical practice.

Chapter 1 begins with an overview of what is normal in terms of health, from two contrasting perspectives of the medical model and social model of health. It then looks at individual, environmental and occupational, political and social influences on health, and considers the World Health Organization (WHO) definition of health.

Chapters 2 and 3 look at how psychology can help explain individual human behaviour in a medical setting. Chapter 2 considers the psychological, cognitive and social dimensions of health and illness and how doctors apply this knowledge to understand and manage patients. Some of the influences on how individuals react and adapt to life events are explored. Chapter 3 looks at psychological models of behaviour and behaviour change and how they can be applied to medical practice.

Chapter 4 moves from the individual to the group or community aspect of health and illness. What sociology is and its importance to medicine are considered with particular reference to fundamental concepts such as structure, culture and community, as well as poverty, ethnicity and gender. The chapter looks at the nature of the doctor–patient relationship and the difference between illness and disease.

Chapters 5 and 6 focus on population health, including differences in healthcare delivery and policy across different parts of the world. Various approaches to measuring and addressing population influences on health, the relevance and practice of epidemiology and some of the factors which influence how disease is treated are considered in Chapter 5.

Chapter 6 builds on the concepts and basics of population health outlined in the previous chapter. Its focus is on supporting positive health through government policy and social change (e.g. health promotion) rather than individual change (see Chapter 3). The chapter includes discussion of the more clinical aspects of public health around the control of communicable diseases in populations, as well as identifying and addressing occupational and environmental influences on health.

Part 2: Applying Knowledge to Clinical Practice

The second part of the book (Chapters 7–9) takes a best practice approach, explaining some of the factors which underpin good, patient-centred clinical care, and applying the knowledge set out in this book to disability and activity limitation, and to community and hospital-based case studies.

Chapter 7 provides an introduction to scientific method and critical appraisal. The chapter looks at how to seek answers to questions that arise in the care of patients and how to achieve best clinical practice. To achieve these aims, the chapter considers the principal research methods, audit and its role in clinical practice, ethics and research ethics, and the role of reflection in practice.

Chapter 8 focusses on disability and activity limitation. Disability is not a case of 'a + b = c'; rather the impact of a limitation on an individual is down to a complex interaction of individual, societal and medical factors. Disability requires a holistic perspective both in terms of understanding what it is like to live with a disability, and how quality of life could be improved, and in terms of working with other professionals to support people with disability most effectively. This chapter also considers very topical issues of quality of life and resource allocation.

Finally, Chapter 9 pulls together many of the aspects of psychology, sociology and population health introduced throughout this book, and applies these to clinical medicine using case studies from community and hospital medicine. It considers how you apply what you know into daily practice, and how you and your patient link into the bigger picture of healthcare.

Learning features

Each chapter follows a similar format with a chapter overview, and the core text followed by a summary and further reading. References are listed at the end of the book. Each chapter begins with setting out the key outcomes addressed in the chapter. Chapters set out why this issue is important and summarise key pieces of evidence. Key issues are explored through case studies (considering the perspective of the medical student or doctor, patient or carer) and activities. Activities include practical tasks with feedback or learning points, critical thinking or research tasks and reflective practice/thinking points. Activities can be carried out by yourself or with others. These are designed to raise awareness, consolidate your understanding of theories and ideas and enable you to improve your practice using models, approaches and ideas.

part 1

The Doctor as a Scholar and a Scientist

chapter 1

An Introduction to Health and Illness in Society

Jennifer Cleland, Shirley Laird and Blair Smith

Achieving your medical degree

This chapter will help you to meet the following requirements of *Tomorrow's Doctors* (2009).

9 Apply psychological principles, method and knowledge to medical practice.

  (a) Explain normal human behaviour at an individual level.
  (b) Discuss psychological concepts of health, illness and disease.

10 Apply social science principles, method and knowledge to medical practice.

  (a) Explain normal human behaviour at a societal level.
  (b) Discuss sociological concepts of health, illness and disease.

11 Apply to medical practice the principles, method and knowledge of population health and the improvement of health and healthcare.

  (b) Assess how health behaviours and outcomes are affected by the diversity of the patient population.

It will also introduce you to academic standards as set out in other documents such as the joint GMC and MSC guidance called *Medical Students: Professional Values and Fitness to Practise* (**www.gmc-uk.org/education/undergraduate/professional_ behaviour.asp**) and the core curriculum for The Scottish Doctor (**www.scottishdoctor. org**) as published by Scottish Deans' Medical Curriculum Group.

Chapter overview

After reading this chapter, you will be able to discuss the following:

* What is normal?
* What is normal in terms of health?

  o the medical model
  o the social model

* Influences on health

  o individual
  o environmental and occupational
  o political and social

* WHO definition of health

What is normal?

Different people use the word 'normal' in different ways. A philosopher views the normal as the most usual. Psychologists and statisticians refer to normal as the middle range of a distribution of values (i.e. statistically normal). A sociologist defines 'normal' as that which is in line with a rule for a particular social or cultural group in society. The *Oxford English Dictionary* defines 'normal' as 'conforming to a standard'. In medicine, 'normal' is often used to mean an absence of physiological pathology (Offer and Sabshin, 1991). In common speech, 'normal' may simply mean 'not abnormal, not strange'!

You will come across 'normal' being used in lots of different ways in medicine. In terms of statistical probability, the mathematical concept of normal distribution means most things being measured are within one standard deviation (the spread of values) in either direction from the mean (the population average or central point). Usually this is taken as 'normal', and is the basis of many measurements commonly used in medicine such as height and weight for age in childhood, IQ (see Figure 1.1), distribution of blood pressure and so on. However, bearing in mind the sociological perspective, measurements of what is normal usually need to be interpreted with reference to group norms. For example, for an adult, a normal resting heart rate ranges from 60 to 100 beats per minute (bpm). For a well-trained athlete, however, a normal resting heart rate may be as low as 40 to 60 bpm. Heart rate is also influenced by age: 120–160 bpm is normal for babies.

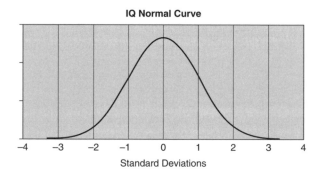

Figure 1.1 IQ distribution.

Source: IQ Comparison Site **www.iqcomparisonsite.com**. Copyright © 2007 Rodrigo de la Jara. Reproduced with permission.

In terms of conforming to a standard, what is considered acceptable behaviour in one population, or social group, may not be seen as such in another group. Dress codes, work habits, gender stereotypes and social intercourse are quite strictly defined in the various cultures of the world and deviation is not generally well accepted. At present homosexuality is seen by most as a normal variation in sexual orientation and sanctioned by law in the UK, for example same-sex civil marriages became legal in 2005. But, in May 2010 in Malawi, a gay couple were arrested the day after their engagement party and jailed for 14 years' hard labour under the country's anti-gay legislation. This example illustrates starkly how different cultural groups have different norms. Figure 1.2 shows a picture of a woman from the Kayan tribe in Thailand where the use of brass rings to elongate the neck (by downward displacement of the collar bones and upper ribs) is thought to enhance beauty. However, she would likely be thought abnormal if seen in a UK city centre.

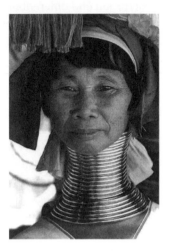

Figure 1.2 Kayan brass rings.

Source: A Kayan woman refugee in Thailand shows her neck rings to sightseers. Author: Steve Evans **www.flickr.com/photos/babasteve/351227116** licensed under Creative Commons.

As a further thought on normality, consider this true experience of a final year medical student. As he travelled by train to an Indian village for his student elective, he thought how abnormal everything was, the people, their culture, the climate and so on. As his journey progressed, he was suddenly struck by the thought, 'It's not all that I'm seeing which is abnormal, it's *me*. I am the one with the different appearance and different cultural background'. Few people regard themselves as abnormal, yet everyone is abnormal to somebody!

What is 'normal' in terms of illness and health? An introduction to the medical and social models of health and illness

There is also a pathological or physiological concept of normality. This 'medical model' defines health as essentially the absence of disease. Using this concept, to 'cure' means to restore a function or organism to a healthy (normal) state or to eradicate illness (abnormality) through diagnosis and effective treatment.

The medical model is driven by the belief that medical science should find cures for diseases in order to return people to health. This model was developed in the nineteenth and early twentieth centuries, and was associated with the discovery of the mechanisms that lay behind infections – specific causes were linked to specific diseases in particular organs, and the task of the physician was to trace the presenting symptoms back to their underlying origins. The era of modern medicine began with the discovery of the smallpox vaccine at the end of the eighteenth century, discoveries around 1880 of the transmission of disease by bacteria, and then the discovery of antibiotics (the sulfa drugs) around 1900.

The medical model emphasises the need to have a good knowledge of biochemistry, pathology, physiology and anatomy in order to diagnose disease. It proposes a scientific process involving observation, description and differentiation, which moves from recognising and treating symptoms to identifying disease aetiologies and developing specific treatments. As such, evidence has always been at the core of the medical model.

With the medical model, informed by the best available evidence, doctors advise on, coordinate or deliver interventions for health improvement (Shah and Mountain, 2007). It is now considered unacceptable to determine treatment on the basis of instinct or 'gut feeling'. Western practice is also increasingly determined by evidence-based guidelines and protocols, with legal consequences for non-compliance.

Development of the medical model enabled biological explanations and treatments for diseases to replace practices based on religious and cultural tradition (e.g. the Greek 'four humors'), which in turn helped to reduce fear, superstition and stigma, and to increase understanding, hope and humane methods of treatment (Tallis, 2004). This was a huge progression. However, the medical model, and its view of normality as absence of disease, has been criticised on many grounds. Firstly, it appears to give doctors a lot of power and patients very little (the paternalistic doctor–patient relationship, see later). This is regarded as outmoded as patients are now seen as experts in their own health, and diagnosis and treatment are often a result of negotiation between doctor and patient (see 'What's the evidence?' below).

What's the evidence?

Breaking bad news

The medical model view of the role of the physician underpinned the development of the authoritarian 'doctor–patient' relationship: all authority over health matters was seen to reside in the doctor's expertise and skill, especially as shown in diagnosis. This meant that the patient's view of illness and alternative approaches to health were excluded from serious consideration. This is known as the activity–passivity, or paternalistic ('doctor knows best'), model of doctor–patient relationships (Szasz and Hollander, 1956; McKinstrey, 1992) now regarded as outmoded. Other models of the doctor–patient relationship have been proposed, such as the guidance-cooperation and mutual participation models. As an example of how these models differ, a doctor who is paternalistic is unlikely to be very concerned with the patient's preferences for treatment whereas this will be very important to a doctor using the mutual participation approach. The role adopted by a doctor depends heavily on the corresponding role adopted by the patient although research shows that, generally, patients are more satisfied with the consultation if they feel you have asked for, and listened to, their views.

Because the major health threats are now not infective diseases but the so-called degenerative diseases (such as heart disease and cancer) and disabling illnesses (such as arthritis and stroke), the medical model is less applicable than was the case when it was first proposed. These conditions are multi-factorial in their development and multi-dimensional in their impact therefore they have neither a simple biological cause nor simple medical or surgical cure.

The medical model also ignores the power of influences other than disease/pathology on health. This is particularly relevant as there is now much scientific evidence that what is considered normal in terms of illness and health may vary by person (individual factors) and by the conditions in which people live (such as living and working conditions). In short, we know now that wider determinants than the presence or absence of disease have an impact on people's health (Dahlgren and Whitehead, 1991).

To summarise, what is 'normal' is very much in the eye of the beholder. 'Normal' in a medical sense is traditionally defined narrowly as absence of disease and/or restoring an organism to normality through eradication of disease. However, changing patterns of disease and mounting evidence that many individual, social and cultural factors influence health have progressed our understanding. While the medical model's scientific, evidence-based approach is core to good medical practice, a broader model of medicine is required nowadays, one which takes into account the vast amount of evidence for influences other than pathology and disease on health.

Social influences on health and illness

In this section of the introductory chapter, we explore some of the influences, other than disease/pathology, on health. These other, myriad influences on health – from population to individual factors – are summarised in Figure 1.3.

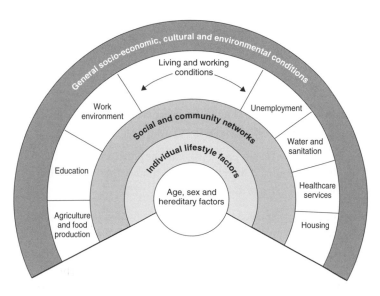

Figure 1.3 Dahlgren and Whitehead's (1991) model of health (Dahlgren, 1991).

This biopsychosocial model illustrates that the chances of a long and healthy life are not the same for everyone. Genetic and constitutional variations ensure that the health of individuals varies, as it does for any other physical characteristic. Surrounding each individual (and their fixed set of genes) are influences on health that can be modified by means other than medical intervention. The first layer is personal behaviour and ways of living that can promote or damage health (e.g. smoking). The next layer is social and community influences. The third layer includes structural factors: housing, working conditions, access to services and provision of essential facilities. To quote the World Health Organization (WHO),

> *The conditions in which people live and work can help create or destroy their health – lack of income, inappropriate housing, unsafe workplaces, and lack of access to health systems are some of the social determinants of health leading to inequalities within and between countries.*
>
> WHO Commission on Social Determinants of Health (2006)

We introduce some of these basic influences on health, and some of the evidence for their importance, in a little more detail below.

Individual influences on health

One individual factor which is highlighted by the model is sex (a biological definition), which can also be construed as gender (a socially constructed role).

The WHO tells us:

> *Gender roles and unequal gender relations interact with other social and economic variables, resulting in different and sometimes inequitable patterns of exposure to health risk, and in differential access to and utilization of health information, care and services. These differences, in turn have clear impact on health outcomes.*
>
> (WHO, 2002)

Gender may influence health status in the following ways:

- exposure, risk or vulnerability (e.g. in women, smoking is linked to lower fertility; men are more likely to develop heart disease)

- nature, severity or frequency of health problems, and the patient's perception of these (e.g. in developed countries, men tend to die younger than women but women tend to report higher rates of illness)

- ways in which symptoms are perceived by the medical profession (e.g. myocardial symptoms are diagnosed later in women compared to men (Mikhail, 2005))

- health-seeking behaviour (e.g. men are less likely to attend the GP)

- long-term social and health consequences (e.g. male patients tend to show greater gains from cardiac rehabilitation than female patients)

ACTIVITY 1.1

Does gender also play a role in *your* education and career?

Does gender influence choice of specialty within the medical profession?

Look at others who work around you – has gender affected their careers?

Another biopsychosocial influence on health at individual level is age. The ability of an organism to stabilise its normal internal environment (body status) is called homeostasis. The homeostatic reserve of the very young and old is less than that of those in early and middle adult life. A good example of this is the more frequent occurrence of delirium with infection at the extremes of the age spectrum. Even influences on the intra-uterine environment can have an effect on health in later life: there is evidence to suggest that low-birth-weight babies are more likely to develop chronic obstructive pulmonary disease (COPD) in later life (see the case study at the end of this chapter). Early upbringing will also influence health in later life. Consider the possible positive and negative effects of childhood diet and exercise, parental smoking and alcohol use, good and bad parenting (and the multiple reasons behind this).

In the elderly population, there is a vast range of what individuals themselves, and society as a whole, consider normal. Many elderly people with multiple pathologies still consider themselves to be normal and healthy by virtue of the fact they can go about their day-to-day lives. Many will also consider significant degrees of joint pain or breathlessness to be a normal part of the ageing process, whereas the reality may be that painful lower limb joints are related to previous sports injuries, arthritis or obesity and that their breathlessness is exacerbated by smoking. Generally, older people see health as functioning even with the presence of chronic disease while young people see health more as fitness (Blaxter, 1990).

Conversely, people with serious physical disability and/or disease consider themselves to be healthy and normal – look at the homepage of Scottish wheelchair athlete, Kenny Herriot (**www.kennyherriot.co.uk**). Sir Steve Redgrave is a rower who won five gold medals in five successive Olympic Games from 1984 to 2000. This was achieved despite having a diagnosis of insulin-dependent diabetes made at the age of 35, a diagnosis of colitis, made just 10 weeks before the Barcelona Olympics in 1992, and lifelong dyslexia.

It seems that adaptation to illness or disability alters the baseline from which the individual judges the nature of health and its implications. In other words, attitude towards health and illness is a relevant individual factor. Health, for many, and for most of the time, is taken for granted and unconsidered for much of the time. On the other hand, being occasionally ill with a cold or flu, or having one or more of the childhood diseases (e.g. rubella, chicken pox), is expected by most people in the UK, and hence is also seen as normal. Similarly, wearing contact lenses or reading glasses is not regarded as being disabled.

These attitudes or lay perspectives influence how individuals respond to symptoms – or health-seeking behaviour. Some people are very sanguine about minor ailments, others rush to the Emergency Department at the first sign of fever in a child. How your mother responded to your childhood ailments is likely to influence how you respond to symptoms as an adult, and as a parent yourself. Work carried out more than four decades ago identified a range of factors which affect the desire to seek professional medical advice. These include: pressure from others, symptoms which are externally visible, symptoms that are perceived to signify serious disease, health beliefs, symptoms which interfere with work and normal functioning (Mechanic, 1968). We will explore many of these factors further in later chapters.

In a similar way that individual or lay perceptions of health vary, so do individual or lay perceptions of risk (see later in this chapter for an introduction to risk). Risk perceptions are people's beliefs, attitudes, judgments and feelings, as well as the wider social or cultural values and dispositions that people adopt, towards hazards. Formal measures of risk include two dimensions – the probability and magnitude of harm. If you think you are likely to be at risk, you are likely to be more motivated to act in such a way to minimise risk. However, people are very good at minimising their own risk. For example, research has shown that family history of lung cancer is linked to objective risk of developing lung cancer but current smokers do not seem to factor this into their risk perception (although 'never-smokers' do), suggesting they minimise (underestimate) their own risk of developing lung cancer (Chen and Kaphingst, 2010).

ACTIVITY 1.2

Think of some unhealthy behaviours you engage in, for example not exercising or smoking. Discuss this with your friends also – what about *their* unhealthy behaviours?

What explanations can you think of for both your own and your friends' behaviours and how do you rationalise your behaviours? What insights might this give you into patients' health behaviours?

Crucial factors in making risk judgments are familiarity, which is about how controllable the risk is, and dread, which is about whether the risk poses a high catastrophic potential. Basically, lay people tend to believe that their chances of experiencing a negative event such as illness are less than average (called 'unrealistic optimism'; Weinstein, 1987). However, they overestimate the frequency of dramatic hazards with low probability (e.g. nuclear power plant accidents) compared to expert risk estimates. They also underestimate high-probability hazards. For example, an obese smoker may think that he is at low risk of premature death from heart disease or stroke because one, or both, of his parents lived until they were into their eighties, although this is actually a high probability hazard for him personally. Lay risk perceptions are also strongly affected by how a problem is presented (see 'What's the evidence?').

What's the evidence?

How data is presented

Lay risk perceptions are also strongly affected by how a problem is presented. The use of medical labelling might cause patients to view themselves as more ill, and hence influence their healthcare behaviour in terms of decisions to seek treatment, how quickly, and whether to comply with that treatment (Young *et al.*, 2008). Media attention or disease mongering may lead to people overestimating their risk of getting a particular disease.

'Disease mongering' is the effort by pharmaceutical companies (or others with similar vested interests) to enlarge the market for a treatment by convincing people that they are sick and need treatment. This works by labelling normal experiences as pathological – for example, 'restless legs syndrome' and 'female sexual dysfunction' have both hit the headlines and become medicalised without research or evidence (Moynihan, 2003). News articles and adverts often exaggerate disease prevalence, are uncritical about data from dubious studies, advocate non-evidence-based approaches, for example fish-oil supplements, and highlight serious consequences of lack of diagnosis and treatment with dramatic, anecdotal headlines (see **www.badscience.net** for further discussion).

As a doctor, or doctor in the early stages of training, identifying and exploring your patient's views of their symptoms/illnesses and how these can be best treated will be time well spent: you can then take their views into account in your explanations and treatment plans.

Environmental and occupational influences on health

The next level of the biopsychosocial model of healthcare is represented by environmental influences on health, including the working environment.

The basic concepts you need to consider when looking at environmental and occupational influences on health are hazards, risks and outcomes.

- Hazard describes the potential to cause harm. A hazard is something that can cause harm if not controlled.

- Risk is a measure of the likelihood of harm occurring from exposure to a hazard. A risk is a combination of the probability that a particular outcome will occur and the severity of the harm involved.

- The outcome is the harm that results from an uncontrolled hazard.

Common hazards (or adverse environmental influences) include the following:

- mechanical (trips and slips, being hit by objects, being injured by equipment)
- chemical (acids, solvents, fumes)
- physical (noise, lighting, vibration)
- biological (bacteria, fungi, blood-borne pathogens)
- psychosocial (stress, bullying, violence from people other than colleagues)

As mentioned earlier, how a person views a hazard depends on their perception of the risk or the expected benefit to be derived from exposure to the hazard. For example, the hazard of smoking is well acknowledged – it causes lung and other cancers, COPD and heart disease, it contributes to many other illnesses and reduces life expectancy and quality of life. The latest figures for 2008 show that around 10 million adults in the UK smoke cigarettes (and this is likely to be an underestimation as it is based on self-report). (See **http://info.cancerresearchuk.org/cancerstats/ types/lung/smoking** for more smoking statistics.) The hazard is appreciated but the risk is not necessarily acknowledged – possibly because of the benefit (pleasure) derived, of other competing needs (peer pressure) or because of underestimating the hazard (it won't happen to me).

Two people exposed to the same amount of a hazard will not necessarily experience the same degree of illness as this is determined by the individual factor of susceptibility. Think back to the social model of health (Figure 1.3) where individual factors, such as genetics, are at the core of the model.

'Harm' generally describes the direct or indirect degradation, temporary or permanent, of the physical, mental or social well-being of workers. For example, repetitively carrying out manual handling of heavy objects is a hazard. The harm/ outcome could be a musculoskeletal disorder or an acute back or joint injury. (Nearly 30 million working days were lost due to workplace injury and ill health in the UK in 2008/09 and back pain was one of the two biggest causes of absence from work [stress being the other].) A general environmental chemical hazard is an air pollutant such as tobacco smoke, leading to a ban on smoking in workplaces and enclosed public places in the UK (**www.smokefreeengland.co.uk**) to reduce the risk of health problems caused by passive smoking. For doctors and other healthcare workers a recognised biological hazard is a needlestick injury, the main risk from which is exposure to blood-borne viruses (BBV) such as Hepatitis B (HBV), Hepatitis C (HCV) and human immunodeficiency virus (HIV). In the workplace, risk may be influenced by complacency – a familiar environment can lead to underestimation of risk. For example, some workers may disregard the need for protective clothing or safety equipment.

It is difficult to compare health and safety in the workplace across countries as health and safety practices and recording systems vary widely. There are also cultural differences in how acceptable it is to report hazards and even workplace injury and/ or death. However, recent media reports of workplace disasters in countries undergoing industrialisation, such as China, are startling.

ACTIVITY 1.3

Work is not all bad. There is much evidence that working is good for your physical and mental health and well-being.

Look up this report and consider the content and the approach taken by the authors Waddell and Burton (**www.dwp.gov.uk/health-work-and-well-being**)

Do you agree with their conclusions?

As discussed above, occupation or workplace is not the only environmental influence on health. Think also about your home, neighbourhood and school/university; the air you breathe and the water you drink; the climate in which you live. The same basic risk factors – mechanical, chemical, physical, biological and psychosocial – are pertinent to the wider environment.

ACTIVITY 1.4

Think about your own environment. Can you identify a list of hazards which you face on a day-to-day basis? Think about where you live, how you travel to university or work (by bike, car, bus or foot), where you spend your day and your leisure time. How do you attempt to minimise any risks (e.g. wearing a reflective jacket and helmet when cycling)?

Historical examples of environmental exposures and health effects include:

- *Cholera* – In nineteenth-century Soho, cholera epidemics were suspected by Dr John Snow to be associated with water supplied by one water company to one pump (the so-called 'Broad Street pump' outbreak). Removing the pump handle stopped the epidemic, leading to the conclusion that cholera was water-borne, before the discovery of its microbiological nature.

- *Air pollution* – In 1952, 4000 people died as a result of severe fog in London. Pollutants from domestic coal burning accumulated in this fog and caused the deaths in susceptible people such as the old, young and ill (particularly those with existing chronic respiratory or cardiac disease). This resulted in the world's first Clean Air legislation (1956), which had a dramatic effect on air quality in Britain's towns.

- *Chernobyl* – A nuclear reactor exploded in 1986 in Russia contaminating over 850,000 individuals with caesium-137. The reactor was encased in concrete and the exposed population monitored, but the true increase in cancer incidence will probably never be known. It is not yet possible to compare this to more recent events in Fukushima, Japan, but there is no doubt that radiation levels will be monitored closely in the long term to assess the impact of this recent disaster.

The London fog example is particularly useful as it highlights the interaction between individual factors (see earlier in this chapter) and environmental influences on health. Climate and weather exert strong influences on health: through deaths in heat waves, and in natural disasters such as floods or tsunamis, as well as influencing patterns of life-threatening vector-borne diseases such as malaria. WHO estimates that environmental hazards are responsible for about a quarter of the total burden of disease worldwide, and nearly 35 per cent in regions such as sub-Saharan Africa. It is clear that poor countries with weak health infrastructure and climatic extremes suffer most from climate and weather influences, and also that weaker individuals, such as the very young and old, and the ill, are most at risk from environmental hazards.

In the context of occupational/environmental influences on health, ill health may be regarded as failure of an individual to be well adapted to his or her environment. This failure of adaptation can be thought of, in simple terms, as the consequence of an adverse environmental influence acting on a susceptible person. Susceptibility is often thought of as simply genetic susceptibility, but this is far from the whole story, since many adverse environmental influences may increase susceptibility to disease (see Chapter 6).

Although it probably seems obvious by now why a doctor practising clinical medicine needs to know about occupational and environmental hazards to health, it is worth setting out some basic points here. If you identify the cause of a disease by taking a thorough occupational/social history, first you have a chance of preventing it in other patients. Second, you should be able to prevent your patient from contracting it again from re-exposure to the hazard. Third, bearing in mind the medical model, it is only from understanding causes of disease that it is possible scientifically, rather than by serendipity, to find a cure or treat appropriately.

The above introduces the wide range of effects that the environment, and the working environment, may have on human health. This will be explored in more depth in later chapters.

Political and social influences on health

Where you live has an enormous influence on your health. On a global scale, infant mortality rates and life expectancy are used as indicators of health. As a rule, poorer countries have the poorest health. In Niger, one of the world's poorest countries, the infant mortality rate is 111 per 1000 live births and life expectancy is 57 years (prediction for births in 2008), although it is currently only 41 years. In the WHO rankings of healthcare systems, Niger holds 170th place. How much is spent on healthcare is relevant to indicators of health: Figure 1.4 looks at spending on healthcare in various countries.

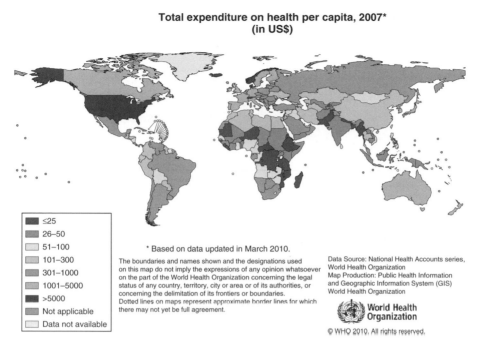

Figure 1.4 WHO comparison of spend on healthcare across the world.

Source: **www.who.int/nha/en**. Reproduced with permission.

On a more local level, it is interesting to look within the UK for examples of how where you live influences health. For example, the poorest areas in Scotland are found in Glasgow. Residence in the deprived areas of Glasgow is associated with increased morbidity and mortality from a range of chronic diseases such as heart disease and lung disease. Healthy food generally costs more than unhealthy food, no matter where you live in the UK, and is also often less available in deprived areas, and this is considered a barrier to good nutrition for people on a low income (Killeen, 1994). To address this barrier, community initiatives have been set up in more deprived areas of Glasgow (and other cities) to improve access to cheap, healthy food.

Countries also differ in terms of effectiveness of healthcare systems. Whilst many reports in the UK media paint a rather gloomy picture of the National Health System (NHS), the British healthcare system remains the envy of many countries across the world. In the WHO rankings of effectiveness of healthcare systems, the UK is ranked 18th despite being ranked only 26th in terms of its per capita healthcare spending. In comparison, the USA is ranked only 37th despite being ranked first in terms of its per capita healthcare spending. Note the percentage of government spending on healthcare (Figure 1.5). In the UK, 87 per cent of healthcare is government-funded, with a very small private sector financed mainly by personal or employer healthcare insurance schemes. This compares, for example, to India where 19 per cent of health-care is government-funded, and the USA (45 per cent).

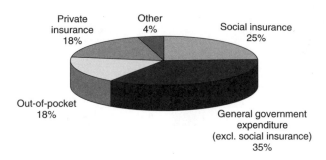

Composition of world health expenditures (world spent US$5.3 trillion on health in 2007)

Private insurance 18%

Other 4%

Social insurance 25%

Out-of-pocket 18%

General government expenditure (excl. social insurance) 35%

Figure 1.5 Government spend on healthcare.

Source: **www.who.int/nha/en**. Reproduced with permission.

The social model of health says that 50 per cent of our health is determined by wider determinants such as where we live, what our income is relative to other people and what level of education we have.

Political and social factors which influence health are not isolated, but interplay in a complex way. For example, research shows that female contraception usage in developed Indian states (e.g. Tamil Nadu) is significantly higher than in less developed states (e.g. Bihar). Both socio-economic status and husband's education are strongly associated with family planning in both states. Religion and caste are associated with family planning in Bihar but not in Tamil Nadu. What explains these differences? It seems that women's education is the key factor: women in states like Tamil Nadu enjoy higher education status and autonomy. On the other hand, women in northern states such as Bihar are strongly subject to traditional conservatism, are predominantly less educated and less likely to work outside their homes. Tamil Nadu has one of the most efficient governance structures in India and the least corrupt state bureaucracy. Bihar, on the other hand, is viewed by many as being misruled.

This example demonstrates the very complex interaction of factors that contribute to health. The link between socio-economic disadvantage and poor health has been demonstrated repeatedly, and across the world (see 'What's the evidence?').

What's the evidence?

A comparative inter-country study published in the *New England Journal of Medicine* (Mackenbach *et al.*, 2008) found that, in all 16 countries included in the study, socio-economically disadvantaged men and women had higher overall mortality rates than did persons with a higher socio-economic status. The universal link between social class and mortality seems remarkable, given the differing disease prevalence and risk factors in these countries. Moreover, relationships between class and mortality are consistent for almost every cause of death.

In summary, in contrast to the medical model, the social model of health places emphasis on changes that can be made in society and in people's own lifestyles to make the population healthier. A broader understanding of the determinants of health also helps to identify what influences health and therefore what can be a barrier to individual and societal health. It is critical to remember that the determinants of health presented in Dahlgren and Whitehead's (1991) model interact with each other. The examples above show how politics influence health but also demonstrate how gender, education and politics can interact in such a way to influence health-related behaviour.

To conclude this section, nowadays in medicine we view the individual as a whole person within a community or society. This leads to any illness or problem being tackled in three ways: physical, psychological and environmental/social. Healing involves more than getting rid of physical illness and, as such, requires a broader definition of health than the medical model.

The WHO definition of health

Moving on from, but not discounting the medical model, we have introduced the wider picture of influences on health. This requires a wide definition of health:

> *Health is a state of complete physical, social and mental well-being and not merely the absence of disease or infirmity. The enjoyment of the highest attainable standard of health is one of the fundamental rights of every human being, without distinction of race, religion, political beliefs or economic and social conditions.*
>
> (WHO, 1948, p. 100)

The WHO definition emphasises psychological and sociological aspects of health, and how these interact with biological processes to create differences in health. This perspective (Schwartz, 1982) proposes that people's social contexts and interpersonal relationships and their perceptions, beliefs and expectations are important factors in the maintenance of health, the development of illness, help-seeking behaviour and responses to treatment.

Using this broader definition of health has implications for how health is addressed. The WHO statement makes very clear that the prerequisites and prospects for health cannot be ensured by the health sector alone – again moving us on from a prevailing medical model viewpoint (i.e. that medical science is solely responsible for returning people to health) to the concept that there are many influences on health, and thus many ways of addressing ill health. The WHO perspective clearly implies that health requires action by governments, by health and other social and economic sectors, by nongovernmental and voluntary organisation, by local authorities, by industry and by the media.

The understanding that health may be considered in more positive terms than just the absence of disease, also lead to the concept of quality of life (QoL). The WHO defines QoL as 'individuals' perceptions of their position of life in the context of the culture and value systems in which they live and in relation to their goals, standard and concerns'. In short, QoL relates to what people see as important in their lives, such as independence and social relationships, as well as physical health. Often relieving physical symptoms will improve a person's QoL but QoL is a complex issue, which may require improving other aspects of the patients' lives such as housing, education, money and relationships. Even in the case of diseases such as cancer, which have a readily identifiable pathological cause, psychological and social interventions and support play a major part in alleviation of distress, discomfort and disability, and therefore in important aspects of health and healing.

We have said above that taking a broader perspective on health than that of the medical model leads to viewing the individual as a whole person, and thus tackling an illness or problem in three ways: physical, psychological and environmental/social. The extent to which each of these three ways will be addressed depends on several factors, including where the patient presents. This is discussed further in the final chapter of this book.

We now introduce Bill, whose story we will follow throughout the book. In this first chapter, we present Bill's social history and a little about his medical history. Different aspects of Bill's disease and symptoms, and their progression over time, will be presented in each chapter.

Case study

Bill is aged 50 years. He works as a payroll administrator in a local bakery firm. He is married to Susan, who works part-time as a cleaner. They live in an ex-council house, which they bought about 20 years ago. They have two grown-up children in their twenties. Their son, Gordon, is married with two pre-school children, lives nearby and depends on Susan for quite a lot of childcare. Their daughter, Tabitha, is at university in Manchester, studying nursing. She comes home during the summers, when she usually works in a local care home to save up some money to eke out her student loan. Bill and Susan try to help her out financially as much as possible but they don't have much spare cash themselves.

Bill has smoked cigarettes (20 per day) since his mid-teens. He doesn't 'do' formal exercise but does like looking after his garden in the summer, curling (a sport in which players slide stones across a sheet of ice towards a target area – look this up in a search engine if you want to find out more) in the winter. Susan makes him lunch to take to work to encourage him to eat a couple of portions of fruit and veg most days – Bill's preference would be to have a pasty and chips in the work canteen! He is overweight, has high blood pressure and high cholesterol and is regularly 'nagged' by his GP to lose weight, do more aerobic exercise and stop smoking. He is resistant to this advice, prefers driving everywhere, and regards generally slowing down and getting short of breath on exertion as normal for his age.

With the introduction of the Quality and Outcomes Framework (QOF) of the General Medical Services contract for general practices in 2004, his GP practice started asking Bill in for regular review of his blood pressure and smoking status. He is always asked if he has considered quitting smoking (to which he mumbles something non-committal, takes the leaflets the practice nurse gives him and then puts them into the bin when he gets home).

A couple of years ago, he was given a lung test (spirometry with reversibility testing). His GP explained that the results of this test indicated that he had COPD, and that this was caused by smoking. Since this diagnosis, he has been invited in annually for a flu jab and was prescribed an inhaler to use every day (tiotropium). He's not quite sure what this inhaler is meant to do but he does take it daily, when he remembers.

Bill doesn't really understand what COPD is – is it the same as emphysema, which his dad had for many years before dying of heart failure at age 63 years? His Dad did smoke but he was a miner, and the doctors said the emphysema was due to being down the mines.

ACTIVITY 1.5

Go to the Cochrane Library (**www.thecochranelibrary.com**) and look up reviews for treatment of COPD. You will see that there are reviews of pharmacological and non-pharmacological (e.g. smoking cessation) treatments. The non-pharmacological treatments – pulmonary rehabilitation and smoking cessation – will be discussed in more detail in later chapters, as will the use of resources such as the Cochrane Library.

Chapter summary

There is more to an ill person than a particular symptom or disease. It is also necessary to consider the person's attitudes towards their health, and the environment in which the individual lives and works. Health may be considered in positive terms, and is related to a global consideration of the quality of an individual's life. By the same token, healing involves more than getting rid of physical illness; it includes an approach to improving or maximising the potential of other aspects of the patients' lives (e.g. psychological, social), and re-establishing 'wholeness' (a word with the Anglo-Saxon same root as 'health'). Therefore, we recognise that to be healthy means more than simply to have no disease but is about a wider concept of well-being. The organisation of healthcare in a country, and broader issues such as level of poverty, education, political stability and environmental factors, which influence both health and healthcare, can all interact as facilitators or barriers to health.

GOING FURTHER

Further reading for this chapter is contained in the rest of the book. Each chapter provides detail on further reading for the particular aspect of health and illness it covers. The references and websites given in this introductory chapter are also relevant further reading.

Useful websites

www.gmc-uk.org/education/undergraduate/professional_behaviour.asp – *Medical Students: Professional Values and Fitness to Practise.*

www.scottishdoctor.org – The Scottish Doctor as published by Scottish Deans' Medical Curriculum Group – Core Curriculum.

www.badscience.net – BAD Science.

http://info.cancerresearchuk.org/cancerstats/types/lung/smoking – Cancer Research UK – Smoking.

www.kennyherriot.co.uk – Kenny Herriot – Scottish wheelchair athlete.

www.iqcomparisonsite.com – IQ Comparison Site – Rodrigo de la Jara (2007).

chapter 2

Using Psychology to Help Your Medical Practice

Jennifer Cleland and Jane Smith

Achieving your medical degree

This chapter will help you to meet the following requirements of *Tomorrow's Doctors* (2009).

9 Apply psychological principles, method and knowledge to medical practice.

   (a) Explain normal human behaviour at an individual level.

   (b) Discuss psychological concepts of health, illness and disease.

   (d) Explain psychological factors that contribute to illness, the course of the disease and the success of treatment.

   (f) Discuss adaptation to major life changes, such as bereavement; comparing and contrasting the abnormal adjustments that might occur in these situations.

It will also introduce you to academic standards as set out in other documents such as the joint GMC and MSC guidance *Medical Students: Professional Values and Fitness to Practise* (**www.gmc-uk.org/education/undergraduate/professional_behaviour.asp**)

Chapter overview

After reading this chapter, you will be able to discuss the following:

- How psychology can help explain individual human behaviour in a medical setting.
- The psychological, cognitive and social dimensions of health and illness.
- How to apply this knowledge to understand and manage patients throughout the life span.
- Some of the influences on how individuals react and adapt to life events, e.g. personality, early experience and resilience.

Psychology applied to medicine

In this chapter, and in Chapter 3, we focus on explaining human behaviour at an individual or psychological level.

In Chapter 1, we gave an overview of some of the many influences on health other than disease/pathology, summarised in Dahlgren and Whitehead's (1991) model of health and the WHO definition of health. This biopsychosocial perspective proposes that people's social contexts and interpersonal relationships and their perceptions, beliefs and expectations are important factors in the maintenance of health, development and progression of illness, help-seeking behaviour and responses to treatment. Understanding your patient's perspective will also inform how you treat and manage that individual patient.

What is psychology?

Psychology is the study of the science of human and social processes and behaviour. It draws on research in the areas of perception, cognition, attention, emotion, motivation, brain functioning, personality, behaviour and interpersonal relationships. Psychological knowledge is applied to understanding and solving problems in many different spheres of human activity, for example health, education and schooling, organisational/industrial, development, personality and social behaviour. Psychology explains normal human behaviour (child development, cognitive and social aspects associated with ageing, normal reactions to life events) as well as providing explanations for different responses to health, illness, disease and other life events (e.g. the impact of having a chronic disease on children's social development, the neurological impact of Alzheimer's disease compared to the normal ageing mind or atypical grief).

In terms of explaining normal human behaviour, the influence of psychology in medicine cannot be underestimated. Some topics from cognitive psychology are presented below to give an overview of the breadth of application of just one area of psychology to being a doctor.

What's the evidence?

Research and evidence from cognitive psychology are used in everyday medical practice. Some examples of this are as follows:

Perception – how information presented by sense organs is recognised

- Visual information – interpretation of scans and radiographs
- Auditory information – using a stethoscope

Attention – the ability to select some information for more detailed inspection while ignoring other information

- Selective attention – focusing on one clinical sign may lead to ignoring another
- Divided attention – looking at a patient's notes on a computer while talking to a patient at the same time

Learning – how performing a particular behaviour is changed by experience

- Skill acquisition – learning to insert a cannula
- Social learning – role modelling in medical education

Thinking – the process of perceiving, classifying, manipulating and combining information

- Decision-making/problem-solving – history taking, making a diagnosis
- Heuristics – using reasoning to make diagnostic decisions

Memory – encoding, storing and retrieving information

- Models of memory and forgetting – apply to learning medicine, swotting for exams, carrying out routine clinical tasks automatically

Language – visual or vocal signals which have meaning to the user and recipient

- Doctor–patient communication, including breaking bad news
- Communicating with colleagues/team working

Stress – experiencing events that are physically or psychologically threatening

- Occupational stress – maladaptive responses to everyday pressures
- Stress management – understand your own response to stress and using effective stress management techniques (e.g. regular exercise, relaxation)

From the Behavioural and Social Sciences Teaching in Medicine (BeSST) Psychology Steering Group 2009 core curriculum for psychology in undergraduate medical education, **www.heacademy.ac.uk/besst**

The examples provided above relate to general aspects of being a doctor but each of these topics also relate directly to patient care. For example, hallucinations and delusions, which characterise psychotic mental illnesses such as schizophrenia, relate to the *perception* of an external stimulus in the absence of any appropriate stimulus (e.g. hearing a voice telling you to behave in a certain way when there is no voice). *Memory* and *learning* are involved in the development of phobias, some of which will (e.g. a hospital, blood or needle phobia), at some point, influence how you plan patient care. *Thinking* and reasoning about health and illness (e.g. deciding whether or not to consult about a particular symptom) is influenced by past experience and learning. Research also shows that health and illness outcomes can be predicted from some enduring characteristics of a person such as *personality* traits and types.

This chapter focusses on two aspects of psychology in medicine. Firstly, we examine how one area of psychology – developmental psychology – can help you understand human behaviour. Age has an important influence on all dimensions of health and affects the aetiology, impact and management of most diseases. This chapter provides an introduction to the associations between age (developmental stage) and health throughout the life span (see Figure 2.1), with the aim of helping you develop understanding, and hence treat and manage, patients effectively. Secondly, we consider how personality and early experience, and how these interact, might influence how a person copes with, or adapts to, stressful situations such as negative life events.

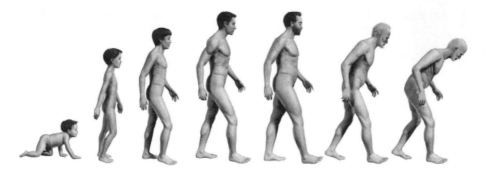

Figure 2.1 Life stages.

Source: Seven Ages of Man © David Gifford/Science Photo Library.

Birth and early childhood

Babies are born with reflexes and behaviours that enable them to respond to the world and develop quickly. Babies come into the world with the ability to selectively respond to humans: they can selectively respond to their own mother's voice immediately (actually even by 24 weeks *in utero*), and their mother's smell within minutes after birth.

How an infant uses the abilities they are born with to underpin physical, cognitive, social and emotional development over the early years of life has attracted much attention from psychologists. The main theorists are Jean Piaget and Lev Vygotsky (cognitive development) and John Bowlby and Erik Erikson (social development). Drawing on the information gathered by these and other theorists and researchers in child development, we now have a detailed profile of normal development. See Table 2.1 for an overview of the key stages in child development.

Table 2.1 Key stages in child development (adapted from Cooper, 1999)

Stage	Approximate age	Key developmental tasks
Infancy	0–2 years	• Forming secure attachment (see later) • Exploring the environment as the basis for sensorimotor, cognitive and social development
Pre-school	2–4 years	Development of basic cognitive and social skills: • Language acquisition • Beginning of autonomy and control • Start of 'Theory of Mind' (how others think) • Moral development around rules • First interactions outside home

Middle childhood	5–11 years	• Intellectual skills
		• Academic achievements
		• Peer relationships
		• Social competence (skills and behaviours for successful social interactions)
		• Emotional competence (understand and respond to own and others' emotions)
		• Gender identity
Adolescence	12–18 years	• Physiological and physical changes (e.g. hormones)
		• Development of coherent self-identity
		• Transition to adult roles and responsibilities, leading to change in family dynamics
		• Development of body image
		• Formation of sexual identity
		• Development of meaningful relationships
		• Independence, autonomy and risk-taking behaviours

What's the evidence?

One of the key tasks for an infant (see Table 2.1) is forming an attachment. Attachment refers to the infant's need to develop a secure relationship with at least one primary caregiver for social and emotional development to occur normally, and it is proposed that further relationships build on the patterns developed in the first relationships.

Research indicates that social, behavioural and mental health problems in later life can stem from early attachment issues. Use 'attachment theory' and 'Bowlby' as key words to search for more information on this topic. Think about factors related to the infant, their caregiver(s) or the living environment that could interfere with forming a secure attachment.

You would have heard of developmental milestones, changes in specific physical and mental abilities (such as walking and understanding language) that mark the end of one developmental period and the beginning of another. Knowledge of age-specific milestones allows parents and professionals to keep track of appropriate development but note that there is considerable variation in the achievement of milestones, even between children with developmental trajectories within the normal range.

Developmental delay refers to delay in reaching important developmental milestones. Developmental delay can be caused by a variety of factors: genetic (e.g. hearing impairment), chromosomal (e.g. Down syndrome), fetal exposure to toxins, peri-natal complications such as birth trauma, and post-natal factors such as malnutrition and neglect. Prevention of, and early intervention in, developmental delay are significant topics in paediatric medicine and clinical genetics. Note that the effects of early influences on lifelong physical health are also becoming more apparent now: the intra-uterine environment may have life-long consequences for adult health. For example, a pregnant woman being overweight or obese means that their future child is more likely to be heavier at birth, and has an increased risk of obesity in adolescent and adult life. At the other end of the spectrum, mortality from chronic obstructive pulmonary disease (COPD) is four times higher in adults who are born in the lowest birth weight group, which is linked to parental smoking. This latter example relates to the 'developmental window' hypothesis, which emphasises the critical importance of early growth and development for subsequent health and disease. Similar, but more complex hypotheses have been developed for other degenerative disease including cardiovascular disease, diabetes and brain development.

Infants grow into children. To work effectively with children, you need to know that they do not just know less than adults, but also that they think differently. For example, young children think things happen just because they have thought or wished it: if a child is angry at one of his/her parents and that parent is hurt or has an accident, the child may feel secretly guilty and responsible for 'causing' the accident because of having 'bad' thoughts about mum or dad. From the point of view of working with children, psychological theory tells us that children are most likely to understand explanations about illness (in themselves or significant others) which:

- take account of their existing level of understanding;

- are linked to their own experiences and immediate concerns; and

- are presented with appropriate non-verbal contextual support (drawings, videos).

As a child matures, they go through a process of transition from vulnerability and high dependence towards autonomy. However, serious ill health can interfere with this process. Psychological research shows that children with chronic illness in general have more frequent psychosocial disturbances than do healthy children of similar backgrounds. Research about children with cancer has found that the chronic strains of childhood cancer, such as treatment-related pain, visible side effects including hair loss, weight gain or loss, physical disfigurement, and repeated absences from school and peers negatively impact on children's social and psychological adjustment. Children with cancer may experience anxiety, behavioural problems, somatic complaints, intense stress, post-traumatic stress disorder (PTSD), academic difficulties and surrounding frustration (due at least in part from school absenteeism resulting from hospitalisation, treatments and treatment side effects), peer relationship difficulties, and worries about the future in relation to career and relationships.

ACTIVITY 2.1

Reflect on possible ways in which having a specific chronic illness (e.g. cystic fibrosis or diabetes) or disability negatively impacts on a child of a particular age to affect their social and psychological adjustment. What factors are likely to influence this? Think about:

- the nature of the condition and its treatment (including the need for hospitalisation), and the limitations and restrictions likely to stem from these
- the age of the child and how the impacts of illness and treatment might affect normal activities of childhood appropriate to the child's developmental stage (as in Table 2.1 above)
- the child's family and wider social environment, including how parents, siblings, peers, teachers and other adults might relate to the child, and cope themselves with any burdens associated with caring for a sick child
- the nature and availability of any support services

How might these factors influence the child's development and maintenance of friendships and other relationships, educational attainment, self-identity, psychological well-being and future prospects? Also think about wider impacts on the family and any potentially positive impacts illness or disability might have on a child or their family.

As a doctor, an understanding that health is more than the absence of disease helps you support the ill child, particularly the seriously and/or chronically ill child and his or her family, through treatment. It highlights the need to involve colleagues and other services, including specialist nurses and psychologists, to help the child and family to develop effective coping strategies and, as far as possible, support involvement in normal childhood experiences which underpin development. Understanding normal development is also important to ensure effective communication with, and assessment of, children. For example, only by knowing about development stages can you assess likely impacts of illness and then work with parents and colleagues to minimise these, 'normalise' their experiences, and know how best to communicate with the child.

Adolescence

Adolescence is the next stage of development after childhood. This is a time of huge physical and psychological change. In terms of the latter, it is useful to know that the key challenges at this stage of development are choosing and adjusting to adult roles, and disputes with adults over rights and responsibilities.

ACTIVITY 2.2

Discuss your experiences of adolescence with other people on your course.

- How did your relationship with your parents change? Do you remember any obvious conflicts?
- How did you work out what was right and wrong for you? You might want to think about risk-taking behaviour such as drinking alcohol or taking drugs.
- Did you always feel as if you fitted in, or did you feel socially awkward or less popular than other people at times?
- How did you cope with the physical changes associated with puberty? Was this a time of hideous embarrassment or were your experiences mostly positive?
- Was it the same for everyone or did individual experiences differ? If the latter, what seemed to help, or hinder, successful adolescence?

Most adolescents get through this time, getting on fairly well with parents and coping with the necessary psychological adaptations, but a significant percentage of them experience problems such as substance abuse, dropping out of school or becoming depressed.

How can psychology help doctors working with adolescents? Firstly, while adolescents have near-adult intellectual ability, neurological development (particularly of the frontal lobes) that continues into adulthood, so adolescents have a greater impulsivity and risk-taking attitude, and poorer impulse control, than adults (Steinberg, 2007). This can have serious consequences in adolescents with chronic conditions such as asthma or diabetes who take up smoking, or who have poor adherence (a huge issue in this group of patients). It is also important to know that adolescents have a strong desire to fit in with their peers and to be considered 'normal'.

However, most adolescents are physically healthy so medical input at this stage of development tends to focus on health promotion and illness prevention, for example reducing use of alcohol and drugs, improving sexual awareness and contraceptive use or interventions to combat adolescents taking up smoking. Medical involvement with those who have difficulties with adaptation tends to focus on treatment of mental health problems or provision of family therapy.

Early adulthood

The period between 17 and 40 years is often described as early adulthood. This is the stage when most people form a lasting relationship, and are focussed on their jobs, marriage/partnership and bringing up children. In terms of psychological influences on health, two aspects of early adulthood have been particularly well researched: the psychology of relationships and having a baby.

There is considerable evidence that men benefit from marriage in terms of physical and mental health, but there is no protective effect of marriage for women. Men tend to also suffer more from the loss of their wives by bereavement or divorce and are more likely to experience physical health problems as a consequence. Sometimes physical symptoms can be a manifestation of marital problems, and recovery from surgery or illness will be impeded by depression following marital separation. Knowledge of the psychology of relationships can help you to understand the context for changes in health and illness: if you suspect this is the case, ask your patient if there are any ongoing family or relationship difficulties as knowing the bigger picture will inform your diagnosis and treatment plan.

Psychological research also indicates that the transition to first-time parenthood is a time of significant change. There are various factors involved in adjusting to the birth of a baby: infant temperament; economic support; quality of spouse support and participation; and parental sex, income, and educational levels are all associated with the ease of this transition. New parents may experience increased exhaustion, loss of sleep, income stress, increased housework, increased worry, decline in sexual relations, increased responsibility, new parenting demands, and a new routine or schedule. Research also has suggested that women may have a more difficult time adjusting to motherhood when parenting expectations exceed their experiences. (It is not all bad; transition to parenthood also may result in benefits such as increased happiness, self enrichment, personal development, family cohesiveness, and strengthened relationships.)

ACTIVITY 2.3

Consider the impact of having a new baby. If you are fortunate enough to have the opportunity to meet or follow a young family as a medical student, knowing a little about the psychological impact of having a new baby, particularly a first child, will help you understand what your patient is experiencing. It is worth exploring the psychological – and physical (e.g. lack of sleep) – demands perceived by the new parent and identifying the ways in which s/he has attempted to adjust to and cope with those demands.

Remember also that parents have a major influence on the psychosocial development of their children (e.g. smoking is twice as likely in children of parents who smoke themselves, how parents react to illness in their children influences how the child goes on to respond to illness as adults) and good parenting is more likely to result in well-developed parenting skills in the next generation. Neglect and physical or sexual abuse are problems that often recur in adults who were exposed as children to these adverse influences.

Generally most people are healthy in early adulthood, and may not have much contact with doctors other than as caregivers to their own children (and perhaps their own parents). This links to the biological factor of homeostasis: a tendency towards stability in the normal body status (internal environment) of the organism. Homeostatic reserve increases during childhood, reaches a plateau in early adult life and declines thereafter. This is the reason why those best able to cope with physical stresses and/or disease are young adults.

Middle adulthood

Different definitions put different limits on this stage, but it is roughly 40 to 65 years of age. There are physical changes at this stage, some of them visible (loss of skin elasticity, greying hair), some less overt (decreased strength and flexibility, declining fertility), and an increase in health problems such as diabetes, heart disease and cancer. Unhealthy lifestyles (obesity, smoking, lack of exercise) tend to catch up with people at this stage as they become less able to react to challenges from the internal or external environment. Many adults become increasingly interested in preventative health at this time, joining gyms and attending for screening (the invulnerability of youth has worn off for many people by this time and there is more awareness of the consequences of one's own actions). As a result, this might be a fruitful stage of development in terms of health promotion campaigns and targeted screening programmes (see Chapter 6 for further discussion of health promotion).

In terms of intellectual ability, fluid intelligence (the capacity to reason and solve problems) has declined with age, but crystallised intelligence (skills and knowledge) increases with age, peaking in middle adulthood (mid-fifties) so the mind is still working well. However, their own parents and children are ageing, and mid-life adults are often caught in between these two generations, becoming caregivers to their parents and having to change caregiving patterns with their adult children.

Old age

Ageing is biological but psychologists and other social scientists highlight that it must be understood in terms of the social environment. How society treats older people influences how they see themselves. Are older people a burden and 'past it' or are they seen as wise and revered? Ageism – 'a process of systematic stereotyping and discrimination against people because they are old, just as racism and sexism accomplish this for skin colour and gender' (Butler, 1987, p. 243) – can be an important influence on how people are treated medically and surgically.

There are obvious socio-cultural differences in how older people are viewed and treated. At the time of writing this chapter, a very small percentage of older people in China lived in nursing or care homes as the cultural norm until recently was to care for one's parents at home, so they are still part of the family and the wider community. This is no longer seen as sustainable given the increasing number of older people in China and the one-child policy, which means there are not enough younger people to look after ageing relatives. Contrast this with the USA, where the social norm for many years for affluent older people is to move to a retirement village or community – especially designed or geared up for people who no longer work, or restricted to those over a certain age. A disadvantage of this set-up is that it adds distance between generations; older and younger people find their friendships primarily within, rather than across, age groups.

Successful ageing depends on many individual and socio-cultural factors, and much research has looked at how best to reduce or delay the onset of impairments that tend to accompany ageing. As with the biopsychosocial model of health (see Chapter 1), the notion of successful and productive ageing is considerably more than the prevention and amelioration of disease. Rather, successful ageing depends on a combination of things, including managing the limitations in physical or other abilities; addressing the negative impact of significant life changes (e.g. retirement, relocation, loss of spouse) on social support and social networks; maintaining and improving performance in those areas that are valued by the older person.

As an example, the older person who anticipates retirement by keeping physically healthy throughout adult life and planning activities (regular golf, holidays, doing a part-time degree programme) to enjoy during retirement; who stays living within easy distance of friends and family; who has a good social network, and who adapts well to loss (e.g. bereavement) is more likely to age successfully, than those who do not have these internal and external resources.

ACTIVITY 2.4

Talk to your grandparents, or older people you are in contact with as a medical student, about retirement. What are/were their goals for retirement? How did they plan for retirement emotionally? Did anything disrupt their plans (e.g. ill health, death of a spouse)? If they have been retired for a while, in retrospect, is there anything they might have done differently?

As mentioned above, bereavement is an increasingly common life event in old age. There has been much research into how people respond to bereavement and other loss, including anticipating their own death or the loss of a relationship. The 'five stages of grief' are often referred to. These are presented in 'What's the evidence' below.

What's the evidence?

The five stages of grief (Kübler-Ross, 1973):

Denial –'This can't be happening, not to me.'

Anger – 'Why me? It's not fair!'

Bargaining –'I'll do anything for a few more years.' The third stage involves the hope that the individual can somehow postpone or delay death or other loss.

Depression – 'What's the point?'

Acceptance – 'It's going to be okay.' In this last stage, the individual begins to come to terms with his or her mortality or other loss.

Kübler-Ross originally applied these stages to people suffering from terminal illness. Later it has been applied to any form of catastrophic personal loss, for example loss of a job, a relationship, of health (such as the onset of a chronic disease, amputation or disfigurement) and also to stages of coping with change.

There is much debate about this model; some research supports it, but other studies have found no evidence for the five stages. However, it can be useful to know that anger, denial and so on are normal reactions to loss, impending loss or major life change, in order to support patients and their relatives.

Kübler-Ross, E. (1973) *On Death and Dying.* New York: Routledge; pages 33–121.

Luckily, research now is focusing more on the health benefits of treatments and interventions in those aged over 65 years of age. For example, physical exercise, in men and women over the age of 65 who had never previously done any formal exercise has been shown to promote cardiovascular fitness. Similarly, smoking cessation can slow down or stop further lung damage or arterial disease even in old age. In terms of cognitive functioning, evidence is accumulating that the adage 'use it or lose it' is appropriate (e.g. frequent participation in mentally stimulating activities is associated with a reduced risk of Alzheimer's disease). As a doctor, it is ageist – and unethical – to dismiss cognitive deterioration in an older person as normal rather than investigating to distinguish normal changes from early signs of pathology.

This is a very general overview of how developmental psychology can help you understand what normal human behaviour is throughout the life span. We have tried to give you some concrete examples of possible ways patients may present at different times in the life cycle, and how major life events like having a baby or being chronically ill might influence individual behaviour. We hope it is clear that even a little knowledge of developmental psychology will help you care for patients in many medical specialties, from child health to medicine for the elderly, general practice and surgical specialties.

Stress and coping

Stress is experienced when the real or perceived demands of a situation outweigh someone's actual or perceived physical, psychological and social resources available to deal with it. Stress is a condition while a *stressor* is the stimulus causing the condition.

Signs of stress can be cognitive (e.g. anxious thoughts, always seeing the worst), emotional (e.g. low mood, tension), physical (e.g. dizziness, chest pain, ulcers) or behavioural (e.g. avoiding the stressful situation). The most common emotional responses to stressors, including those related to illness and its impacts, are anxiety and depression. Anxiety and depression may require attention (treatment) in themselves, but also because of the effects they can have on coping with illness and its treatment (discussed further in Chapter 3).

Coping is any action which is carried out to alleviate stress. The two key figures in this field, Lazarus and Folkman (1984), define coping as 'constantly changing cognitive and behavioural efforts to manage specific external and/or internal demands that are appraised as taxing or exceeding resources.' Specific coping responses are the behaviours, cognitions and perceptions in which people actively engage to deal with life problems.

To help explain people's responses, similar actions are sometimes grouped together as different 'coping strategies' (Skinner *et al.*, 2003). These cover:

- problem-solving, involving direct action, decision-making or planning;

- support seeking, covering social support, comfort and help seeking;

- escape-avoidance, including disengagement, denial and wishful thinking;

- distraction, involving finding alternative activities to do; and

- cognitive restructuring based on positive thinking and accommodation.

Coping strategies are also sometimes further classified as (1) 'emotion-focussed', aimed at modifying the response to a problem, and sometimes referred to as palliative, avoidant or defensive coping, and (2) 'problem-focussed', involving action to change and address the stressor, also referred to as problem-solving or approach coping. Usually a range of coping strategies is important to meet different challenges, in different situations and at different times. Situations in which something constructive can be done (e.g. help-seeking, taking action) will favour problem-focussed coping, whereas those situations that simply must be accepted (e.g. being ill) favour emotion-focussed coping (see also Chapter 3).

Personality

We now turn to considering some of the variables that might influence how a person responds or adapts to stressful situations such as negative life events. Research shows that how people respond to events, and health and illness outcomes, can be predicted from some enduring characteristics of a person such as personality. Psychological factors which explain the varied responses of individuals, groups and societies to disease that contribute to illness, the course of the disease and the success of treatment, including behavioural change and treatment adherence, are discussed in the next chapter.

Personality is used to describe the constellation of attitudes, temperament and character that most satisfactorily distinguishes people as unique individuals. These characteristics are present from late childhood, are relatively enduring traits and are distinct from symptoms such as depression or emotional states that are transient (Taylor *et al.*, 2003, p99).

Personality type refers to the psychological classification of different types of individuals. Carl Jung was the first to propose the notion of personality types in the 1920s. Jung's view was that individuals are either born with, or develop, certain preferred ways of thinking and acting. Possibly the best-known assessment tool of Jungian personality type is the Myers-Briggs Type Indicator (MBTI) (**www. myersbriggs.org**). The MBTI sorts psychological differences into categories with a resulting 16 possible psychological types. None of these types are *better* or *worse*, they are just different. Jung's personality type theory has been criticised, as has the MBTI itself, but it is widely used for team building, career guidance, professional development and leadership training.

You may have heard of Type A and Type B personalities. Impatient, achievement-oriented people are classified as Type A, whereas easy-going, relaxed individuals are designated as Type B. The theory originally suggested that Type A individuals were more at risk for coronary heart disease but this claim has not been supported by empirical research, rather it appears that one particular dimension of the Type A personality, labelled 'hostility', is a risk factor.

Most researchers now believe that it is impossible to explain the diversity of human personality with a small number of discrete types so trait models of personality are more popular now.

One trait model of personality is that of the 'big five' personality dimensions of neuroticism, extraversion, openness to experience, agreeableness and conscientiousness. Studies examining the association between personality traits and studying medicine have found that preclinical performance is predicted by conscientiousness, one of the 'big five' personality dimensions (Ferguson *et al.*, 2003). Individuals with high conscientiousness see themselves as practical, thorough, and hardworking, rather than disorganised, lazy, and careless, and so it is perhaps not surprising that such individuals do better in preclinical examinations. A number of studies and meta-analyses have confirmed the predictive value of the Big Five across a wide range of behaviours.

Whichever approach one takes, personality basically relates to the fundamental emotional and behavioural characteristics of a person. Personality is thought to be innate but personality interacts with environmental factors, and indeed certain genetic factors may predispose an individual to interact with, or respond to, his or her environment in a certain way. For example, research indicates that underlying temperament (personality) not only can set the stage for an eating disorder to manifest, but will also act as a catalyst for its maintenance. Thus, the influence of environment, particularly early environment, on personality has implications for coping with life as an adult.

How personality and early experience interact

Psychological factors such as personality and early experience contribute to illness, the course of the disease and the success of treatment. These are discussed briefly in relation to two key phenomena – the development of resilience and the development of attitudes towards health and illness.

The development of resilience

Everyone experiences major life changes – a little brother or sister being born, starting school, school exams, leaving home to go to medical school, starting work, starting a new relationship, and so on. These examples could be broadly seen as positive, but most of us also experience bad life events – the death of a close family member, being ill, losing a job, the end of a significant relationship, long hours or lots of pressure at work.

ACTIVITY 2.5

In an attempt to measure life changes, Holmes and Rahe (1967) developed the Life Events Scale (also known as the Social Readjustment Rating Scale, or SRRS). The life events are ranked in order from the most stressful (death of spouse) to the least stressful (minor violations of the law). Look for the SRSS online (**www.psychlotron. org.uk/resources/physiological/AQA_AS_stress_srrs.pdf**) and work through it in terms of events in the past year of your own life. This will give you a rough estimate of how stress might be affecting your health. If you score 300, you may wish to consider seeking support.

Holmes, TH and Rahe, RH (1967) The social readjustment rating scale. *Journal of Psychosomatic Research* 11(2): 213–218.

Any sort of change can make you feel stressed, even good change. Most people going through major life changes can expect to feel varying levels of shock, anger, anxiety, stress, confusion and possibly self-doubt (e.g. 'have I made the right decision?'). It's not just the change or event itself, but also how you react to it that matters. What's stressful is different for each person. For example, one person may feel stressed by retiring from work, or going to university, while someone else may not. How shock, anger, anxiety and/or stress are expressed also differs by individual. Some people cry, others do not. Some people get angry ('why me?'), others do not. There is no right or wrong way to cope with change, but there are ways which are more adaptive than others. These include talking to others, exercising, looking after oneself, trying to anticipate difficulties in order to have action plans to deal with difficulties, and so on.

Sadness, and having good and bad days, is part of a normal adjustment, or response, to life events. Depression, or denial, and not being able to cope with normal life activities are not; these are sometimes called maladaptive responses. Adaptive or normal adjustment to life events means that feelings of grief, anxiety, stress, confusion and self-doubt should not become persistent, but should decrease over time. For example, people who are bereaved should feel better over time, and while how long this might take is different for different people, most people who lose someone close feel better within a year or two.

Research has identified variables that influence how an individual copes with major life events: sudden loss is more difficult to adjust to than expected loss; social support and connecting to others, including talking to a professional, is also known to be an important factor. Individual factors are very important; some people are more resilient than others. 'Resilience' is the positive capacity of people to cope with change, stress and adversity. For example, you will know people who seem to cope well with failing an exam at medical school. These are the people who, soon after the initial shock, accept the situation and work towards changing it (i.e. studying for the resit). Other people don't take it so well. They blame others (e.g. the questions were too hard, the simulated patients were unrealistic), get angry or depressed, and don't accept that their summer plans will need to change so they can study for the resit. The first example is someone who is resilient, who can cope with stress and adversity, the latter less so.

Resilient people adapt successfully to change or challenges. This adaptation may result in the individual 'bouncing back' to a previous state of normal functioning, or using the experience of exposure to adversity to grow stronger (much like an inoculation gives one the capacity to cope well with future exposure to disease).

Resilience is best understood as a process rather than solely an individual personality trait. In this sense, 'resilience' occurs when there are cumulative 'protective factors'. Certain protective factors contribute to resilience, particularly early life experiences such as good parenting/positive childhood experiences, which can in turn underpin the development of self-confidence/self-esteem, social support, and good problem-solving skills. For example, in terms of problem-solving skills, resilient people might plan for change more effectively than people who are not resilient. If you take the example of going to university, thinking of potential difficulties (e.g. missing your family) can help you plan how to cope with them (e.g. choosing a university which has good transport links with your home town).

Most research now shows that resilience is the result of individuals interacting with their environments and the processes that either promote well-being or protect them against the overwhelming influence of risk factors. These processes can be individual coping strategies, or may be helped along by good families, schools, communities and social policies that make resilience more likely to occur. In my specialty (Liaison Psychiatry: JC), I see a lot of people with very negative childhood experiences such as sexual abuse and poor parenting, who have gone on to develop either clinically significant psychiatric problems or just do not have the coping skills to manage daily hassles, let alone major life events, effectively. Of course, I never see the people with equally difficult upbringings who manage well, who are resilient. These individuals have had sufficient protective factors (such as individual traits, or positive school experiences) to manage life effectively and to respond to life events adaptively.

The development of attitudes towards health and illness

Evidence suggests that the adult response to illness is the product of a process that begins in childhood. Illness behaviour refers to any behaviour in response to illness, for example, taking medication or a day off work. Illness behaviour is often labelled as negative (abnormal or maladaptive) or positive (normal or adaptive). Examples of each are addiction to analgesia (maladaptive) and attending rehabilitation classes (adaptive).

That illness behaviour is based on social learning (i.e. learning from others) beginning in childhood is suggested by empirical research. Studies show that levels of illness behaviour are higher for adults who recall being encouraged to adopt the sick role as children (reinforcement) or whose parents had high levels of illness behaviour (modelling).

What's the evidence?

A study using videotaped parent–child interactions showed that, in comparison to adolescents who coped well with chronic pain, adolescents who did not cope well with chronic pain had mothers who were significantly more likely to exhibit behaviours (such as complaining about pain) that discouraged the adolescent's efforts at coping with an exercise task (Dunn-Geier *et al.*, 1986).

Similarly, Rickard (1988) found that children of chronic lower back pain patients exhibited a higher frequency of behaviours (e.g. more complaining, more days off school, more visits to the school nurse) hypothesised to be learned through observation of and interaction with a chronic lower back pain parent than children of diabetic or healthy parents.

Dunn-Geier, BJ, McGrath, PJ, Rourke, BP, Latter, J and D'Astous, J (1986) Adolescent chronic pain: the ability to cope. *Pain*, 26: 23–32.

Rickard, K (1988) The occurrence of maladaptive health-related behaviours and teacher-rated conduct problems in children of chronic low back pain patients. *Journal of Behavioral Medicine*, 11: 107–116.

Results of these and similar studies provide support for a social learning perspective on the development and maintenance of sickness behaviour in children. We will discuss the idea of social learning further in the next chapter.

ACTIVITY 2.6

Stop and think about how your parents responded to your illness as a child and how you now respond to illness as an adult. Then think about any families you might have seen in general practice or in paediatrics. How were the parents responding to illness in their child – by fussing or by supporting the child in a calm manner?

Related to illness behaviour is the idea of the 'sick role', a term discussed in more detail in Chapter 4.

Case study

Bill, our 50-year old patient with COPD, has said to you that he wishes his disabilities were more evident as he feels negatively judged for having a disabled parking permit but looking healthy enough through the eyes of the naïve observer. He also feels to blame for having COPD as it is due to smoking. He is also aware that his dad died young and smoking probably contributed to his death. He seems to be getting quite down about things, is not coping terribly well with being ill, but at the same time seems to be quite accepting of slowing down and symptoms such as shortness of breath and nasty chest infections.

What psychological factors might be influencing how Bill views having a chronic illness?

Chapter summary

This chapter gave a brief overview of how psychology can help explain normal human behaviour. The chapter focussed on two aspects of psychology in medicine. First, how developmental psychology, including pre-natal influences, can help you understand human behaviour. Second, we considered how personality and early experience, and how these interact, might influence how a person copes with, or adapts to, stressful situations such as negative life events and illness. You should now be able to discuss:

- how psychology can help explain individual human behaviour in a medical setting,

- the psychological, cognitive and social dimensions of health and illness,

- how to apply this knowledge to understand and manage patients throughout the life span, and

- have an appreciation of some of the influences on how individuals react and adapt to life events.

GOING FURTHER

Edwards, M and Titman, P (2010) *Promoting Psychological Well-Being in Children with Acute and Chronic Illness*. London: Jessica Kingsley Publishers.
This book discusses issues such as the impact of diagnosis, the experiences of children and their families in managing their medical condition and treatment, and strategies to support children and help them to cope with medical conditions.

Robbins, PR (2007) *Coping with Stress: Commonsense Strategies*. Jefferson, NC: McFarland and Co Inc.
This book covers the nature of stress, and which methods of coping seem to be effective and which do not.

Useful websites

www.gmc-uk.org/education/undergraduate/professional_behaviour.asp
www.myersbriggs.org

chapter 3

The Interaction of Psychological Factors with Illness, Disease and Treatment

Jane Smith and Jennifer Cleland

Achieving your medical degree

This chapter will help you to meet the following requirements of *Tomorrow's Doctors* (2009)

9 Apply psychological principles, method and knowledge to medical practice.

(c) Apply theoretical frameworks of psychology to explain the varied responses of individuals, groups and societies to disease.

(d) Explain psychological factors that contribute to illness, the course of the disease and the success of treatment.

(e) Discuss psychological aspects of behavioural change and treatment compliance.

(g) Identify appropriate strategies for managing patients with dependence issues and other demonstrations of self-harm.

It will also introduce you to academic standards as set out in other documents such as the joint GMC and MSC guidance called *Medical Students: Professional Values and Fitness to Practise* (**www.gmc-uk.org/education/undergraduate/professional_behaviour.asp**).

Chapter overview

After reading this chapter, you will be able to discuss the following:

* The importance of an individual's behaviour and other psychosocial factors, including stress and emotions, in the promotion of health and avoidance of self-harm, and in the prevention, presentation, treatment and management of illness.
* How psychological models of behaviour and behaviour change can be applied to medical practice.
* The role of doctors, multi-disciplinary team members and different types of intervention in contributing to psychological aspects of care.
* How to apply this knowledge to understand and manage patients.

This chapter discusses how psychology can be applied in medicine to aid understanding of the health and illness experiences of individuals and families. The above learning outcomes from *Tomorrow's Doctors*, expanded to represent how they will be discussed here, essentially cover the many ways in which psychological factors such as behaviours, cognitions (thoughts) and emotions, and social factors operating at the individual level interact with health, illness and disease. The main pathways by which these interactions occur, which will be used to structure the chapter, are shown in Figure 3.1.

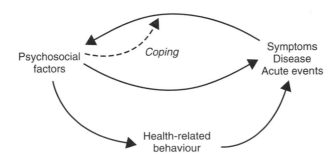

Figure 3.1 Interactions of psychosocial factors with illness.

That the mind and body interact, and that psychological factors play a role in illness and disease is evident in situations where people's lifestyles, behaviour and other psychological characteristics are seen to contribute to ill health. It is also illustrated when people present with ill health without a physical cause, or when two individuals with the same underlying impairment experience dramatically different levels of disability and outcomes. As per the biopsychosocial model described earlier (see Chapter 1), the interaction of biological, psychological and social factors in health has implications for medical practice, including:

- recognition of more individual responsibility for patients in the prevention of ill health and treatment and management of disease;

- the need for treatment of the whole person, and not just a disease;

- recognition of there being no clear distinctions between health and illness, and the importance of the patient's perspective in defining ill health;

- consideration of psychological factors as causes as well as consequences of disease.

Health-related behaviour

People's behaviour in relation to their health, or 'health-related behaviour', is important in terms of:

- primary prevention of disease and the promotion of health in healthy individuals;

- secondary prevention of ill health, that is in ensuring that people experiencing health problems recognise and present with symptoms appropriately so that they can be treated in a timely fashion to avoid worsening of a condition or complications;

- treating acute conditions, where appropriate 'sick-role behaviour' (see Chapter 4) is important in facilitating effective and speedy recovery or rehabilitation;

- ongoing chronic disease management, where there is increasing emphasis on patients sharing responsibility with health professionals for managing their condition, which involves them engaging in 'self-care' or 'self-management behaviour'. The terms self-care and self-management are often used interchangeably but self-care is sometimes used more broadly to also refer to actions taken by individuals to look after themselves (e.g. self-medicate) in the face of minor illness.

ACTIVITY 3.1

What do you do on a day-to-day basis to keep physically and mentally healthy?

Several key health-related behaviours serve as important behavioural risk factors for the development and progression of a range of common chronic conditions. These, and the main conditions in which they have a causal role, are shown in Table 3.1. Changing some of these behaviours is an important target for treatment of several conditions (e.g. physical activity as part of rehabilitation for cardiovascular disease, COPD and diabetes). Attendance at regular appointments, adherence to medications, self-monitoring (e.g. of blood pressure, blood sugar, peak flow) and avoidance of factors which may exacerbate the condition are additional self-management behaviours common across a range of diseases. In individuals who are both healthy and ill, ensuring adequate sleep and hygiene practices are also important on a day-to-day basis for keeping well.

Table 3.1 Key behavioural risk factors for chronic diseases, definitions linked to recommendations and diseases to which behaviours are linked

Behavioural risk factor	Definition	Major diseases linked
Smoking	= any regular/prolonged	• Cardiovascular diseases (e.g. high blood pressure, coronary heart disease, stroke) • Chronic obstructive pulmonary disease • Some cancers (esp. lung, mouth, throat)
Overweight/obesity	= BMI >25 (overweight), >30 (obese), abdominal fat	• Cardiovascular diseases • Type 2 diabetes • Some cancers

Poor diet	= high saturated fat = low fibre, fruit and veg (< 5 portions/day) = high salt = high red/processed meat, low fish	• Obesity • Type 2 diabetes • Cardiovascular diseases • Some cancers (esp. colorectal)
Lack of physical activity/sedentary behaviour	= <30 mins moderate intensity activity on 5+ days/week, <20 mins vigorous intensity activity on 3+ days/week or equivalent	• Obesity • Type 2 diabetes • Cardiovascular disease • Osteoporosis • Back pain • Some cancers (esp. colon, breast)
Excessive alcohol consumption	= >14 units for women, >21 for men, binge drinking = 6 units for women, 8 for men on one occasion	• Obesity • Liver disease • Cardiovascular disease • Some cancers (esp. liver, mouth, esophageal, bowel, breast) • Diabetes • Osteoporosis • Pancreatitis • Psychiatric disorders

Engaging in risky behaviours can be thought of as deliberate self-harm (DSH). In emergency medicine (A&E) and psychiatry, DSH tends to refer to self-injury, often by self-cutting or deliberately taking an overdose, and is usually associated with psychiatric disorder such as depression, schizophrenia, borderline personality disorder and substance misuse. However, other colleagues and specialties have a much broader definition of self-harm: as engaging in harmful behaviours – or not behaving in certain ways (e.g, not exercising). Think of a middle-aged, male patient with obesity, high blood pressure and high cholesterol, a smoker with a family history of heart disease who does not follow recommended treatment and lifestyle advice – taking the broad view, this patient could be considered as demonstrating self-harm. Working with patients with self-harming behaviours involves applying the approaches discussed in this chapter – behaviour change and self-management techniques, and psycho-education.

Factors influencing health-related behaviours

A range of biological (genetics, age), environmental (availability, access), social (culture, class, education, support) and enduring psychological factors (past and concurrent behaviours, personality) influence people's engagement in healthy and unhealthy behaviours to varying degrees. For example, there is evidence that alcoholism has a strong hereditary component, availability of cheap fast food is implicated in poor dietary practices and obesity and most health-related behaviours show a socio-economic gradient whereby the lower social classes and poorly educated are more likely to engage in unhealthy behaviours (smoking, poor dietary practices, physical inactivity). Many of these factors and enduring psychological characteristics (personality) are difficult or impossible to change, particularly within the remit of normal medical practice. Thus, most efforts to change people's health-related behaviours focus on targeting specific social and cognitive determinants of behaviour. Psychological models or theories provide suggestions on how best to do this.

Models of health-related behaviour and behaviour change

One of the earliest models, developed specifically in the context of influencing people's health-related behaviours as part of early US public health campaigns in the 1960s, is the Health Belief Model (Becker, 1974). This postulates that beliefs that a person holds about their health and the behaviour in question, along with possible cues to action, prompt people's health-related behaviour. For example, when applied to smoking, the model suggests that someone who believes that:

(1) they are susceptible to getting a smoking-related disease (lung cancer, COPD), perhaps because of age or family history,

(2) the disease has severe consequences,

(3) the benefits or pros of giving up (saving money, better health) outweigh the cons or barriers (short-term withdrawal symptoms, weight gain) and

(4) who is generally motivated to improve their health

would be more likely to give up smoking than someone who does not hold one or more of these beliefs.

People's beliefs about the nature of their illness, and a balance of their perceptions about the necessity (pros) of their medication and the concerns they have about it (cons), has been shown to explain medication-taking across a range of conditions. However, beliefs only explain a small amount of the variability in people's actual behaviour. A number of other psychological factors have been shown to be important also, and some of these are incorporated into the Theory of Planned Behaviour (TPB; Figure 3.2, Ajzen, 1985). The TPB provides more detail on how a wider range of beliefs combine to influence people's behaviour. These are as follows.

(1) Attitude, reflecting a positive or negative evaluation of the behaviour based on what are believed to be the consequences of the behaviour and how important they are.

(2) Subjective norm, representing people's beliefs about significant others' views on the behaviour and how important it is to comply with those views.

(3) Perceptions of control over their behaviour, reflecting beliefs about internal and external factors which make the behaviour easier or harder to perform or change.

In turn, these attitudes, subjective norm and perceived control influence people's behaviour via their effects on people's intentions to perform or change their behaviour. For example, a person would be more likely to decide to lose weight if they:

- hold a positive attitude towards weight loss;

- believe it would bring about consequences that are important to them (e.g. looking better, improved health);

- believe people important to them think they should lose weight;

- feel they have the necessary resources, skills or opportunities to overcome barriers to losing weight.

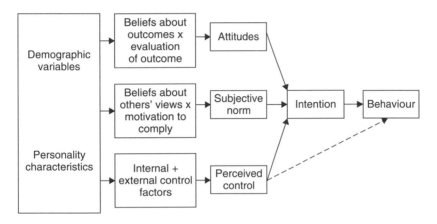

Figure 3.2 Theory of planned behaviour.

Source: Ajzen (1985). Reproduced by permission of Professor Icek Ajzen.

The Theory of Planned Behaviour recognises the importance of social factors acting on the individual, for example peer pressure. Research using the model also highlights that, as we know from common experience, people's good intentions about their health-related behaviour do not necessarily translate into action. Why not? This 'intention–behaviour gap' seems to be linked to perceived control over the behaviour.

Perceived control is similar to a concept shown to be important in influencing people's health-related behaviour, and indeed behaviour in general, known as *self-efficacy* (Bandura, 1977). Self-efficacy is the belief that one can perform a novel or difficult task, or cope with adversity. Perceived self-efficacy facilitates goal-setting, effort investment, persistence in the face of barriers and recovery from setbacks. A healthcare example would be believing you can lose weight, sticking to a diet even when it is difficult to do so and not giving up the diet when you have a blow-out.

ACTIVITY 3.2

The General Self-Efficacy Scale (GSE) was created to assess a general sense of perceived self-efficacy with the aim in mind to predict coping with daily hassles as well as adaptation after experiencing all kinds of stressful life events. Higher scores mean higher self-efficacy. Try the GSE for yourself.

Table 3.2 The General Self-Efficacy Scale

1 I can always manage to solve difficult problems if I try hard enough.
2 If someone opposes me, I can find the means and ways to get what I want.
3 It is easy for me to stick to my aims and accomplish my goals.
4 I am confident that I could deal efficiently with unexpected events.
5 Thanks to my resourcefulness, I know how to handle unforeseen situations.
6 I can solve most problems if I invest the necessary effort.
7 I can remain calm when facing difficulties because I can rely on my coping abilities.
8 When I am confronted with a problem, I can usually find several solutions.
9 If I am in trouble, I can usually think of a solution.
10 I can usually handle whatever comes my way.

1 = Not at all true 2 = Hardly true 3 = Moderately true 4 = Exactly true

Source: Schwarzer and Jerusalem (1995). Reproduced by permission of Dr Ralf Schwarzer. **www.ralfschwarzer.de**

Self-efficacy has also been proved to be important in long-term maintenance of behaviours (e.g. maintaining adequate physical activity, a healthy diet). This links self-efficacy to the idea that behaviour change is not a one-off event but can be seen to proceed in a number of stages, during which different psychological factors and processes may be important. Several stage theories have been proposed to capture this, the most widely researched of which is the Stages of Change or Transtheoretical Model (Prochaska and DiClemente, 1984; see Table 3.3).

ACTIVITY 3.3

Thinking about your current levels of physical activity and recommended levels of activity for maintaining health (30 minutes of moderate-intensity activity, such as brisk walking, on 5 or more days of the week, or 20 minutes of vigorous-intensity activity, such as jogging, on 3 or more days of the week), which stage from the Stages of Change model are you in (see Table 3.3)?

Table 3.3 Stages of Change

Stage of Change	Description	Example
Precontemplation	Not yet acknowledging that there is a problem behaviour that needs to be changed.	I currently do not exercise and do not intend to start in the next 6 months.
Contemplation	Acknowledging that there is a problem but not yet ready or sure of wanting to make a change.	I currently do not exercise but I am thinking about starting to exercise in the near future.
Preparation	Getting reading to change.	I currently do some exercise, but not regularly.
Action	Changing behaviour.	I currently exercise regularly, but have only recently begun doing so.
Maintenance	Maintaining the behaviour change.	I currently exercise regularly, and have been doing so for some time.
Relapse	Returning to old behaviours and abandoning the new ones.	I usually exercise regularly but my exercise has recently slipped.

Source: adapted from Prochaska & DiClemente, 1984

If you would like to increase your physical activity, think about how you might address psychological factors that influence your behaviour, in light of the models above.

Models such as the Stages of Change model are used every day in medical practice, in general practice (e.g. smoking cessation) and chronic disease management (e.g. diabetes clinic), and, in particular, in the field of addictions/dependence. The Stages of Change model shows that, for most people, changing addictive or otherwise maladaptive illness-related behaviour takes place gradually. They move from being uninterested, unaware or unwilling to make a change, to considering a change, to deciding and preparing to make a change. Determined action takes place after a period of contemplation, preparation and often after failed attempts at change, sobriety or abstinence. Relapses can take place along the way. It is easiest to think of this in relation to a clinical example such as smoking cessation. Guidelines state that GPs and other health professionals should offer opportunistic smoking cessation advice at every appropriate opportunity. In one appointment, the patient may be quite certain they do not want to quit. However, when the same patient comes in a few months later, they are more open to discuss this, and seek cessation support (e.g. nicotine replacement therapy) from the GP. The same patient may quit successfully for many months but then resume smoking at a time of stress, only to start the cycle of change again in the future.

ACTIVITY 3.4

Can you think how you would use behaviour change theory when working with a patient who is dependent on alcohol? This particular patient knows he has an alcohol problem and can see the benefits of giving up, but cannot see how the short-term difficulty would be outweighed by the long-term gains.

You may also want to draw on the other psychological theories presented in this chapter to help you explore your patient's cognitions and emotions about their difficulties and the possibility of change.

In summary, people's beliefs about the nature of illness and its threat, the pros and cons of performing a behaviour, their positive or negative attitudes towards the behaviour, beliefs about what others think and their motivation to comply, and self-efficacy appear to be important to address in motivating people to change their behaviour, and forming an intention to act. It is also important to know that people are not always ready to change, but can move through stages, from not wanting to make a change to action, or from changed behaviour to a relapse (e.g. resuming smoking).

Stress, emotions and health

The above models all assume that people make rational decisions about their health-related behaviour and focus on the need to alter people's cognitions or thinking to facilitate changes in their behaviour. Although these are important, as Chapter 2 describes, stress and emotional factors are also frequently shown to be related to health-related behaviours, for example, in terms of symptom perception.

The self-regulatory model (Leventhal *et al.*, 1992; see Figure 3.3) highlights that there are complex interactions between cognitions and emotions which influence people's responses in the face of ill health in terms of whether, for example, they seek help, take medication or perform behaviours to actively manage their condition. The different types of coping referred to in the model are presented in Chapter 2.

There is growing recognition that stress and its ensuing emotions can also contribute to ill health and disease independent of their effects on people's health-related behaviour.

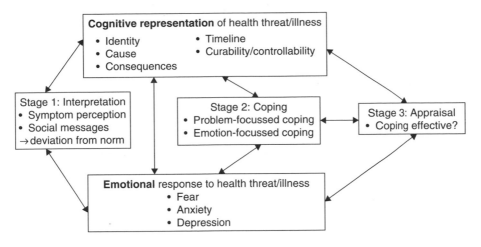

Figure 3.3 Self-regulatory model.

Source: Adapted from Ogden (2007) and Leventhal *et al*. (1992).

ACTIVITY 3.5

Using the self-regulatory model, think about an asthma patient experiencing a respiratory symptom. Consider how different cognitions about the symptom and/or asthma as an illness (top box in Figure 3.3), the patient's emotional state (bottom box) and perceived ability to cope with the symptom (middle box) might interact to influence their symptom perception. In turn, how might this feed back to affect subsequent cognitive and emotional responses and their actual action to deal with the symptom (details of coping are covered later)? What might be the consequences?

Symptom perception

In those with an existing diagnosed physical problem (e.g. asthma), symptoms with a psychological cause (e.g. hyperventilation due to panic) can be misattributed to the illness, increase reported morbidity, and potentially lead to unnecessary escalation of treatment (e.g. overuse of reliever inhalers) with possible side effects and further morbidity. Furthermore, a significant proportion of people present with physical symptoms which are not tied to any underlying pathology. Such 'medically unexplained symptoms' can represent expression of psychological problems through physical symptoms, a process known as somatisation. Irritable bowel syndrome is an example in which gastro-intestinal symptoms suggest a problem with the function of the gut, but no abnormalities in structure are found.

When patients present with medically unexplained symptoms, serious organic causes must obviously be eliminated. However, if the potential importance of psychological factors is not recognised and carefully acknowledged, the patient may undergo endless unnecessary investigations and referrals, potentially reinforcing their concerns about having a serious physical disease, reducing their satisfaction with the doctor–patient relationship and contributing to an increasing cycle of chronic illness and disability.

Remember that symptoms without an identified physical cause are no less 'real' than symptoms with an identified pathology. Indeed, psychological factors play a role in patients' experiences, perception, interpretation and reporting of all *symptoms*. This is most clearly illustrated and best understood in the context of pain. A common definition of pain as 'an unpleasant sensory or emotional experience associated with actual or potential tissue damage or described in terms of such damage' acknowledges that emotional as well as sensory processes are inherent in the experience of pain. There are descending neural pathways in the spinal cord, by which signals from the brain linked to cognitions and emotions, can modulate incoming sensory signals from the site of pain. This can explain the potential for negative emotions to worsen pain, placebos that patients believe will work to reduce pain, and cognitions related to the cause and meaning of the sensations to influence perceived levels of pain, or indeed whether the sensation is experienced as pain at all! Indeed, in clinical practice, you will hear colleagues refer to pain as 'in the eye of the beholder', which is just another way of saying pain is a subjective experience.

Stress response and disease processes

Psychological factors can also affect the development and progression of disease, independent of their influence on health-related behaviours or symptom perception, due to the physiological effects of stress on bodily systems (think about your physiology teaching and learning, and the 'fight or flight' response). When a stressor is psychosocial and does not necessitate physical action, the stressor is prolonged, or bodily systems are already weakened, the response can have detrimental effects on various bodily systems, including components implicated in disease pathophysiology.

The area where this has been best researched is in relation to cardiovascular disease. For example, sympathetic nerves and stress hormones can act on the cardiovascular system to increase blood pressure, heart rate response, heart size, clotting, atherosclerosis, vasoconstriction and pro-inflammatory cytokines and can lead to arrhythmias, endothelial dysfunction and altered metabolism. Chronic stress therefore has potential to contribute to the development of cardiovascular disease in healthy individuals, especially in a subgroup of people who respond to stress with high cardiovascular reactivity. Thus, cardiovascular disease illustrates that both illness itself, and the consequences of illness, can be viewed as stressors (see Chapter 2), placing demands on a patient.

In the medical model, diseases and their consequences are defined in terms of mortality and objective measures of morbidity related to abnormalities in biochemical, physiological or physical functioning. However, situations where there is a mismatch between people's apparent or reported subjective disability and ill health and clinical measures of disease severity (which can happen, for example, when the situation outweighs the patient's capacity to cope, i.e. stress) highlight the need to take a more holistic view of the illness experience from the patient's perspective.

As Figure 3.4 illustrates, assessments of the subjective impacts of illness at each of these more complex levels captures not only the direct impacts of any underlying disease or disorder, but also the way in which psychological and social factors increasingly influence a patient's perception, management and evaluation of these. For example, for two given children with asthma of a similar severity assessed via a measure of inflammation or respiratory function, the levels of symptoms (e.g. breathlessness) reported may vary according to their psychological state or their interpretation of the meaning of the symptoms. The extent to which these symptoms then affect their ability to undertake physical activity might depend on whether they have taken treatment or how accustomed they are to feeling breathless. Furthermore, whether any limitations lead to them reporting reduced well-being or quality of life would be influenced by their evaluation of the importance of the activity to them, for example whether they actually want to be able to do sports or doing so has social implications. The figure also illustrates that sometimes an impairment (e.g. facial scarring) may not in itself result in any disability or limitation, but can still cause handicap or restrictions in functioning (e.g. embarrassment restricting social activities). Disability is discussed further in Chapter 8.

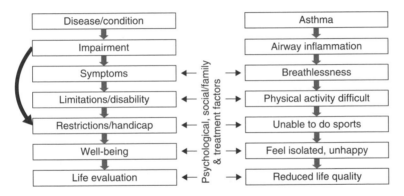

Figure 3.4 Levels at which subjective impacts of illness can be assessed.

Source: Adapted from WHO (1980, 2002), **www.who.int/classifications/icf/en**

Various outcome measures have been developed to assess patients' subjective experiences of specific symptoms, health-related quality of life, general quality of life and so on (see **http://phi.uhce.ox.ac.uk** for examples). These usually attempt to tap into people's perceptions of various dimensions of well-being including physical (e.g. symptoms, mobility), psychological (e.g. cognitive, emotional) and social (e.g. social activities, sexual functioning) aspects. These measures are increasingly used in clinical practice to identify and prioritise problems that might be overlooked if traditional clinical measures of disease impacts alone are used, aid communication and incorporate patient preferences around decision-making in relation to treatment, and monitoring response to treatment from the patient's perspective.

Psychological impact of disease

The most common emotional responses to stressors, including those related to illness and its impacts, are anxiety and depression, both of which can affect the illness
itself and treatment (see also Chapter 2). However, in physically ill patients, anxiety
and depression may be missed as such symptoms might be disregarded as part of
the illness, and many formal measures used to assess anxiety and depression cannot
distinguish ambiguous physical symptoms resulting from the anxiety and depression
from those stemming from an underlying illness. The Hospital Anxiety & Depression
Scale (Zigmond and Snaith, 1983) is often used for screening for and assessing severity of anxiety depression amongst physically ill patients because it does not rely on
assessment of physical symptoms.

Depression has been shown to be more common in life-threatening or chronic
illness, where there is unpleasant or demanding treatment, when a patient has
low social support or lives in adverse social circumstances, or has a prior history of
depression, alcoholism or drug abuse. It may also be a side effect of treatment, or
a direct consequence of neurological damage in some conditions (e.g. in stroke).
Again, if prolonged, recurrent or severe enough to interfere with functioning or
treatment, depression requires formal assessment and management. This is because
research suggests that anxiety and depression across a range of diseases may
subsequently result in poor adherence and self-care, self-destructive behaviours
and detrimental effects on disease processes (as for chronic stress). This in turn can
lead to reduced survival, increased risk of further acute events and complications,
increased symptoms, disability and reduced quality of life, prolonged recovery and
poorer outcomes from treatment, and increased costs of care.

Figure 3.5 provides guidance on when and how to intervene in patients presenting with depressive symptoms alongside physical illness.

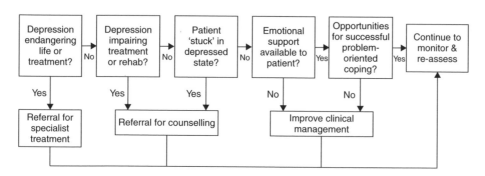

Figure 3.5 Dealing with depression in patients with chronic illness.

Source: Salmon (2000). Reproduced with permission by Wiley-Blackwell.

It must also be remembered that in assessing and discussing illness experiences
and patients' responses to them, the impact of any illness is not a one-off experience.
Patients' responses to impacts develop and change over time as they go through a

process of coping and adjustment, and face new challenges in the course of their illness. There are similar processes, or normal stages, of adjustment after diagnosis of a chronic illness or diagnosis of a life-threatening/fatal illness and bereavement (see discussion of the stages of grief in Chapter 2). Such frameworks are somewhat simplistic as these processes are not necessarily linear, but they can provide a further means of assessing adjustment, providing reassurance regarding the normality of a patient's experience, and guiding the need for and timing of intervention/information if patients appear to get 'stuck'.

Thus, illness, its many impacts in different domains and the challenges it presents in the form of disruptions to daily living, treatment and hospitalisation, uncertainty and threat to future and the burden of ongoing self-care and lifestyle changes can be viewed in terms of stressors (see also Chapter 2). These stressors place demands on patients and families, requiring them to respond and adapt. Adaptation is achieved via responses at physiological and psychological (behavioural, cognitive and emotional) levels and coping is the process in which a patient or family actively manages stressors in an attempt to reduce the perceived discrepancy between the demands a stressor places on them and the resources they have available to deal with it. A range of coping strategies is important to cope with illness and illness-associated stressors, in different situations and at different times, for example in terms of dealing with an acute event (e.g. hospitalisation) in the course of illness, as opposed to ongoing management of a condition. It may not be possible to directly address some problems (e.g. death of a family member, diagnosis of a chronic condition), in which case emotion-focussed coping is the only option, and may be helpful in the short-term to deal with the shock and initial extreme emotions experienced.

ACTIVITY 3.6

What specific coping strategies do the following actions represent? With reference back to Chapter 2, pages 36–37, what type of coping (emotion- or problem-focussed) do they reflect?

1. Setting goals for gradually building up activity after a heart attack
2. Self-discharging from hospital after an asthma attack on insistence that well
3. Finding out information about ways to improve diet
4. Seeking alternative therapies instead of drug treatments
5. Practising relaxation exercises prior to surgery
6. Exercising to exhaustion to prove recovery post-myocardial infarction
7. Refusing help from others despite difficulties with tasks
8. Seeing self as better off than others because you survived
9. Continued heavy drinking on belief that nothing will help
10. Talking to other patients about illness

As Activity 3.6 illustrates, in practice some coping strategies (e.g. seeking support) can be problem- or emotion-focussed depending on the purpose served (e.g. emotional support, or practical support to deal with a problem), and strategies may overlap and be co-dependent.

There may be limitations on a patient's ability to cope and this may be influenced by illness-related factors (e.g. the level of threat to life/functioning, side effects of treatment), background personal factors (e.g. personality, socio-demographics, timing in life, knowledge, previous experience) and physical or environmental factors (e.g. financial resources, social or family support).

In terms of developing your own medical practice, the doctor often has a key role in helping patients cope in terms of forming a supportive relationship. This can include providing opportunities for disclosure, effective listening, and ensuring continuity and follow-up, and also facilitating support where necessary by, for example, involving others (e.g. referral to the community mental health team) and facilitating access to formal programmes and/or the support groups that exist for many conditions.

Psycho-educational interventions and support

Patients with chronic disease may be referred to formal programmes, such as cardiac or pulmonary rehabilitation or self-management education to improve their coping skills and strategies. Such programmes, especially for cardiac and COPD patients, often include exercise to improve functioning, reduce anxiety about exertion and promote positive well-being. They also usually include education about the disease, its treatment, self-management, and lifestyle changes and adherence necessary to reduce disease progression and complications. As a result of typically being provided in a group setting, provision of social support and involvement of carers is common. Programmes also sometimes include stress management, for example via relaxation training, and psychological techniques to facilitate behaviour change by addressing some of the key social and cognitive factors influencing behaviour highlighted above (e.g. to enhance self-efficacy, address beliefs, facilitate goal-setting). There may also be psychological assessment and treatment for emotional problems, although this is variable across different diseases. For example, in multi-disciplinary pain management programmes and interventions to support coping with musculoskeletal conditions such as rheumatoid arthritis, attention is often paid to patient's emotional well-being and how they are coping with their condition. It would be interesting to compare and contrast the outcomes of these holistic programmes with those which focus solely or primarily on promoting medication adherence and performance of behaviours central to medical management of the conditions (Newman *et al.*, 2004).

A generic 'expert patient' self-management programme led by trained lay people has also recently been implemented in the NHS to support people in managing a range of chronic diseases (**www.expertpatients.co.uk**). This addresses issues common across numerous conditions such as symptom recognition and management, lifestyle changes, self-management and adherence, stress, and communication with health professionals. The initiative links to increasing emphasis on the need for 'partnership' between patients and health professionals in chronic disease care.

It is not possible here to discuss in detail provision of rehabilitation, self-management education, specific psychological interventions or other multi-disciplinary programmes and care for specific conditions. However, a first port of call for summaries of evidence on the effectiveness and key components of such programmes and important aspects of primary and secondary medical care related to providing psychological and educational support to patients are disease-specific management guidelines (**http://guidance.nice.org.uk/Topic**, **www.library. nhs.uk/guidelinesfinder**). The Cochrane Library is a collection of systematic reviews of trials of a range of specific interventions across many conditions (**www. thecochranelibrary.com**).

ACTIVITY 3.7

Think about Bill, the COPD patient used as a running case study in this book. Look up relevant management guidelines (**http://guidance.nice.org.uk/Topic**, **www.library. nhs.uk/guidelinesfinder**) and conduct a search of the Cochrane Library to identify what is recommended with regard to psychological aspects of care for patients with COPD. How would this impact on your practice, and courses of action: (1) as a GP, and (2) as hospital doctor in light of his presentation at the end of Chapter 2?

Case study

As Bill's GP, you are becoming quite frustrated with his passive acceptance of his COPD symptoms. You know that smoking cessation would help halt the deterioration in his lung function while increasing physical activity would improve his general health and fitness. You decide that your first step is to ask him to book a double consultation so you can explain to him the difference smoking cessation and exercising would make to his general health. You plan to 'sell' this to him by linking this to growing old healthily as you think that should be important to everyone.

Is this approach, which is based solely on your own beliefs about health, likely to work?

How could you use psychological theories of health behaviour and health behaviour change to encourage and support him to stop smoking and take up gentle exercise?

Chapter summary

You can draw on the framework and models presented in this chapter to better identify, understand, consider and address psychosocial issues interacting with illness, disease and treatment to improve care for individual patients. Communication with patients about psychosocial issues needs to strike a balance between dismissing their importance and potentially making patients feel helpless and victims of circumstances beyond their control, versus attributing entire responsibility to patients and making them somehow feel to blame for their suffering. It is then important to consider each of the pathways by which psychosocial factors interact with illness by doing the following:

1. Identifying and attending to patient's appraisal, coping and adjustment to disease impacts, especially enduring emotional problems and the need for social support.

2. Addressing psychosocial factors potentially impacting directly on disease process and symptoms, via 'stress' management.

3. Providing education and support for patients in changing relevant health-related behaviours, with due consideration of key social-cognitive determinants of behaviour change (e.g. beliefs, self-efficacy) and the skills, techniques (e.g. planning, goal setting, monitoring) and resources to implement and maintain changes.

Where difficulties are encountered, patients may require referral to specialist multi-disciplinary teams, which increasingly have members with relevant psychological expertise (e.g. psychologists, liaison psychiatrists, trained specialist nurses), or specific psycho-educational programmes and services.

GOING FURTHER

Ogden, J (2007) *Health Psychology: A Textbook.* Berkshire: Open University Press.
   This book provides a comprehensive review of theory and research in health psychology, and gives details of behaviours such as smoking, exercise and eating.

Useful websites

www.gmc-uk.org/education/undergraduate/professional_behaviour.asp

http://phi.uhce.ox.ac.uk

http://guidance.nice.org.uk/Topic

www.library.nhs.uk/guidelinesfinder

www.thecochranelibrary.com

chapter 4

The Sociology of Health and Illness

Maureen A. Porter and Edwin van Teijlingen

Achieving your medical degree

This chapter will help you to meet the following requirements of *Tomorrow's Doctors* (2009)

10 Apply social science principles, methods and knowledge to medical practice.

   (a) Explain 'normal' behaviour at a societal level.
   (b) Discuss sociological concepts of health, illness and disease.
   (c) Apply theoretical frameworks of sociology to explain the varied responses of individuals, groups and societies to disease.
   (d) Explain sociological factors that contribute to illness, the course of the disease and the success of treatment – including issues relating to health inequalities, the links between occupation and health, and the effects of poverty and affluence.
   (e) Discuss sociological aspects of behaviour change and treatment compliance.

This chapter introduces some of the key concepts in the sociology of health and illness. It will help you develop an understanding of what sociology is, and its relevance to medicine and medical practice. It should encourage critical thinking about concepts which are often taken for granted in medical care as well as the role of evidence-based medicine.

Chapter overview

After reading this chapter you should be able to understand:

- What sociology is and what kind of issues it addresses.
- Fundamental sociological terms such as structure, culture and community.
- The nature of the doctor–patient relationship and culturally competent care.
- The difference between illness and disease, and that becoming ill is a social as well as a biological process.

What is sociology?

Sociology aims to understand the social world and the way that individuals fit into it. We all live in societies, or groups, constrained by laws and customs and interacting with each other on a daily basis. Some of these societies are rich and well governed with adequate provision of schools, jobs and hospitals. Others are poor or war torn; women and children live in fear of rape or murder and few people have shelter, clean water or sufficient to eat. The way that people act and interact in society cannot be divorced from the context of their lives.

In the past, sociology was described as the 'science of society' because it uses scientific methods – surveys, interviews, observation and documentary analysis – and theory based on empirical evidence, to explain patterns of human behaviour. For example, why do children from poorer families (a particular group) do less well at school than those from better-off families? In answering this question, the sociologist might focus on the sorts of parental support typically available to children in such families or the attitudes towards education prevailing in the playground. Psychologists, in contrast, would be more interested in how individual children might respond to parental incentives or encouragement. Thus, both sociologists and psychologists attempt to explain the observed pattern of behaviour, and perhaps to change it for one more beneficial to society and the individual, but they work from different theoretical and conceptual stances.

In addition to studying society at this *macro* level, sociologists also study it at the *micro level* of human interaction. Within the wider society, most of us live and work in smaller groups like families, communities and teams. We are members of leisure organisations, occupational groups (e.g. 'medical student') etc., where we interact with others, talking and building social relationships and understandings. Sociologists start from the assumption that we are social actors who interact with one another and our environment and in so doing shape the world in which we live.

Bearing this in mind, sociology defines what is 'normal' as that which is in line with a rule for a particular social or cultural group in society at a particular time. A micro level example of this would be taking for granted as we grow up that we will one day marry and have children. Whether or not we are married, many people succeed in having children, but the unexpected experience of infertility can lead to questioning our assumptions about our bodies, relationships, families and medical treatment. Couples to whom this happens can suffer psychological problems and cut themselves off from the world of 'normal' people and 'parents' to avoid confronting the shame and hurt of being childless.

ACTIVITY 4.1

The sociological perspective of health is concerned with factors in the outer layers of Dahlgren and Whitehead's (1991) (see Chapter 1) model of health – social and community networks, general socio-economic, cultural and environmental influences. Consider how these factors could contribute to asthma in Kai, a four-year old child.

Kai lives in a rented flat with his mother, Fiona. The flat is very small and smells of damp. His mum does not work, she is a single parent with no family nearby, so she has to be available to look after him most of the time (he is at nursery only two afternoons per week). They live on benefits. Fiona does not have a car so she has to shop locally. This is quite expensive and the range of healthy food is very limited. Finally, they live in quite a built-up area with only one small park within walking distance.

As well as trying to describe and understand the social world, sociologists also try to explain it, developing theories or adopting perspectives from other contexts such as philosophy or history. The complex relationship between a manual worker and his white collar boss for example can be explained in many different ways depending on one's theoretical perspective. A *Marxist* (someone who believes in changing and improving society by implementing socialism) might see it as one of exploitation, the boss bullying the worker to produce goods he does not own and perhaps never can, for the capitalist boss who profits from his labour. A *functionalist* (someone who sees society in terms of the function of its constituent elements, namely, norms, customs, traditions and institutions) might take a more conciliatory stance, seeing both as working at their different capacities to produce a product whose sale will benefit them directly, and indirectly the rest of society (e.g. through the tax system). If the boss is a man and the worker a woman, then *feminists* (whose focus is establishing and defending equal political, economic and social rights and equal opportunities for women) might add to these analyses the issue of gender politics, the exploitation of women by men mimicking the sexual hierarchy of the wider society.

An example which is pertinent to medicine is the sociology of professions. There are two contradictory theoretical perspectives in the sociology of professions (see MacDonald, 1995, for an overview). In the older of the two perspectives, professions represent the institutionalisation of altruistic values, since the professionals are seen as committed to providing services for the common good. Thus teachers, lawyers and doctors differ from stockbrokers and company directors in that the former occupations consist of people who are not directly motivated by personal interest, nor by financial gains. The latter occupations consist of people working for an immediate economic gain. Those engaged in a profession are often said to have a vocation, *a calling*.

Sociologists who studied professions in the 1950s drew up a list of characteristics of professions as opposed to other occupations (Greenwood, 1957).

1. Systematic theory

2. Authority recognised by its clientele

3. Broader community sanction

4. Code of ethics

5. Professional culture sustained by formal professional sanctions

Medicine incorporates all the above features. It has a (1) theoretical basis; (2) patients come to doctors for advice/help, and also governments come to the medical profession for advice/help; (3) no one is allowed to practise medicine without a licence; (4) Hippocratic Oath, etc.; and (5) strong professional organisations that guard the quality of the work done by its members.

More recent sociological thinking approaches the idea of professions from the notion of 'power and control' (Klegon, 1978). Such theoretical approaches stress *competition* between different occupations. The crucial feature of the division of labour in healthcare is seen as the control that doctors exercise over their own work and that of allied occupations and patients. The maintenance of the medical profession requires the continuing exercise of power and control over allied and competing occupations. From this perspective, the function of nurses, for example, can be seen as to serve the doctor and maintain the power dynamic that privileges medicine over nursing. This dominance in terms of power and control may be threatened by extended roles and scopes of practice for allied professionals (e.g. nurse and pharmacist prescribers), and government policy changes (e.g. reduced length of training for hospital specialties).

What is important to remember is that the sociological theories used to explain behaviour are not right or wrong. They all contain elements of truth and may help us to understand the situation better, albeit from a particular standpoint. Thus, sociology also provides theoretical frameworks to explain how individuals, groups and societies interact and respond to situations.

Fundamental sociological concepts

Several concepts are particularly important to sociology because they are fundamental to describe the social world and social interaction. Knowing a little about these concepts will help you understand the position of a group of patients, or an individual patient from a particular group in society, and consider what sociological factors may contribute to their presentation, response to treatment, etc. Furthermore, thinking about people as members of groups is helpful in terms of working with colleagues from different healthcare professional groups, and even different groups or specialities within medicine (e.g. surgeon, paediatrician, general practitioner).

This section provides brief explanations of the fundamental sociological concepts of:

- Social structure
- Culture
- Community
- Ethnicity

Social structure is a result of the way a society is organised and is also part of its functioning. For example, social class is a structure which operates at the individual level by affecting the opportunities available and the way of interacting with the world and at societal level by redistributing wealth and scarce resources.

Social institutions such as political parties, schools, marriage and families, hospitals, the church or the mosque are part of the structure of society. They differ from one society to another but serve much the same purpose. Such institutions developed historically to maintain social order but continue to be revised and updated as society evolves. For example, in the 1960s it was shameful for a child to be born outside marriage in Britain; recently it was estimated that more children will be born to unmarried parents than married in the very near future, reflecting a changing attitude in British society towards the institution of marriage.

Culture has many meanings but is generally used to convey the ethos of a society, the way that the structure interacts with the people living in that society. Hence many Western societies produce what is usually called 'high culture', i.e. opera, theatre, poetry, ballet and representational art. In India, by contrast, music and dance take different but no less sophisticated forms. But the term 'culture' also refers to the use of language between individuals – what is acceptable and what is not varies from society to society, from group to group (see also Chapter 1) – and to conventions for behaviour or manners. For example, the behaviour of a football crowd shouting abuse at the referee and other team is tolerated in the setting of the stadium whereas shouting abuse is not usually acceptable in other contexts. Often groups develop a way of thinking, dressing or speaking, which reflects their difference from the rest of society as in 'youth culture' or 'drug culture'. Some ethnic or religious groups are said to have a culture which promotes and values formal education, so the culture is conducive to educational experience (e.g. Asians), whereas other cultures do not (e.g. Caribbean). It is useful to be aware how cultures can be reflected in the behaviour of various groups. At the same time, however, generalisations by group can lead to stereotyping so caution must be applied in labelling any one group or culture as one thing or another.

ACTIVITY 4.2

Think about your own culture. Can you identify a list of factors which help others to identify you as being part of one particular community or separate from another? Think about how you live, how you present yourself in different situations and environments, your family traditions. How many communities can a person belong to at the same time? Someone can be a student, a parent with a child at the local primary school, Irish, Protestant, a poet, a lesbian and a Mancunian all at the same time.

In healthcare, different professional groups have very different cultures. For example, in the past, nursing was viewed as having a culture of blame and punishment in response to patient safety errors (e.g. suspended from duty). With clinical governance, however, there is less differentiation between individual healthcare professions, and the culture of patient safety has moved to a system-wide approach around error management. Thus, we have moved from a blame culture to one of system change and education.

What's the evidence?

'An organisation with a memory', published by the Department of Health in 2000 (**www.dh.gov.uk/en/Publicationsandstatistics/Publications/PublicationsPolic yAndGuidance/DH_4065083**), reviews the scale and nature of serious failures in National Health Service (NHS) healthcare, to examine the extent to which the NHS has the capacity to learn from such failures when they do occur and to recommend measures which could help to ensure that the likelihood of repeated failures is min- imised in the future. The report talks about organisational culture change as key to learning from and preventing failures in safety.

Community is a central concept because within most societies there are many different communities which may be defined as people grouped according to some attribute which they have in common. In Britain today, there are Muslim communities and Jewish communities (i.e. defined by religious beliefs); there are black and white communities (ethnicity), working class and middle class (social class) and farming or retail communities (occupation). People do not need to live together to be part of a community though they should identify with that group in some way. For example, British people living abroad often have little in common but their origin and are widely dispersed, yet they form what is often referred to as an 'expat community', using the same language and often sharing the same values. There are some communities – such as housing estates – which are defined by geography as well. The elderly in a care home along with the staff caring for them might be seen as forming a community, as might all those in a 'cottage hospital' but a large teaching hospital would probably not consti- tute a single community. Geographical areas are often defined as 'communities' for the purpose of policing though they may have no more in common than a shared locality.

It is immediately obvious that individuals will often belong to more than one community. Black working class women are likely to live in certain neighbourhoods (location), they belong to an ethnic group (culture), and they are part of the working class as well as women (both social stratification). White Anglo-Saxon Protestant (WASP) pensioners in an American suburb also belong to different communities, some of which might or might not overlap with the black working class women. Nei- ther is being part of a community static. In reality, we see that people move between different communities during their lifetime (e.g. teenage community is a commu- nity based on life stage). People move physically from one area to another, but they might also move from one social group to another, or from one functional group into another (e.g. from students to doctors or from being members of a students' union to being members of a trade union) and people might be socially mobile within the social stratification. Thus, a medical student brought up in a working class family in a rural area might move to become part of the urban middle classes as he/she becomes a doctor and moves to an urban area.

The main points to bear in mind are that 'community' can mean something dif- ferent to someone else, and people can be part of different communities at the same time. Generally, community implies a sense of belonging.

Social capital is a term used to define what resources individuals bring to their lives, connections and experiences which they can fall back on when necessary. If you think about financial capital as money which can be used when necessary, to build a new school or hospital or fund a health education project, the same can be applied at the individual level. Your own financial capital enables you to buy a new computer should your current one break down tomorrow. In other words, it is not used for everyday activities but cushions the blow of not having a computer to do your work at home tomorrow. Social capital is similar in that it can cushion an individual at times of social or health need, allowing him or her to draw on resources such as friends and family relationships. One frequently quoted definition is that of Bourdieu (1986, p. 248) who argues that social capital is 'the aggregate of the actual or potential resources which are linked to possession of a durable network of more or less institutionalized relationships of mutual acquaintance or recognition'.

There is some evidence that those with access to 'social capital' in the form of more and better social networks, such as their family, friends, neighbours, colleagues at work and active memberships of organisations and good social relationships with people in those networks tend to do better in life. They seem to cope better with austerity and have goodwill available within their networks upon which they can fall back if necessary. Hence active older people looked after in their own homes or those of close relatives tend to live longer, healthier lives than those confined to care homes or institutionalised in hospitals. Social capital also works the other way, the individual is the source of social capital for his or her friends when they are in need of extra support. Organisations such as the National Childbirth Trust and MumsNet increase the social capital of mothers with dependent children, providing them with support, emotional and physical assistance at a time when they can be feeling isolated and vulnerable.

The term 'ethnicity' refers to social groups who share a cultural heritage with a common language, values, religion, customs and attitudes. The members are aware of sharing a common past (unlike the members of many communities), possibly a homeland and experience a sense of difference. 'Race' is often treated as interchangeable with ethnicity but usually refers to physical characteristics such as skin colour, hair type and facial features. Unemployment is higher among most ethnic minority groups than in the indigenous population and results in poorer housing, poverty and inequalities in health (Senior and Bhopal, 1994). Ethnicity and health are discussed in more detail later in this chapter.

By studying the social structures, cultures and communities of groups of people in all parts of the world, sociology attempts to understand and explain how society is organised and how individuals in these different societies experience life. It has many branches or topics of interest including industry, religion, family, sport, education, media, sexual divisions or deviance, and medicine.

Why sociology is important to medicine

Sociological concepts and theories are useful for explaining relationships between many different social factors such as the relationship between social class, wealth and health. People in richer countries tend to enjoy better health and to live longer lives than those in poorer countries although the best health is found in societies where the gap between the wealthiest and the poorest is least, such as Sweden.

Basically, the lower down the social class the more ill health there is, and the sooner people die. This is referred to as the health gradient. This could be due to *poverty*, people being unable to afford a good diet or to live in damp-free housing or feeling safe enough outside to take exercise. They may not be able to use health services effectively because of the cost of travel or an inability to take time off work for healthcare. There is evidence that health facilities are less common in depressed areas than in affluent, a situation dubbed by Tudor Hart (1971) as 'the inverse care law'. It could also be due to *poorer working conditions*, heavy manual labour in an unhealthy environment or unemployment making life more dangerous. The stress of such work may lead people to seek solace in unhealthy substances such as alcohol and tobacco. It could be the result of *educational differences*, people not knowing what constitutes a balanced diet or how to live a healthy lifestyle. All these factors are outside patients' direct control, which means that it may not be easy for the doctor to help the sick patient as he or she cannot change their life situation and circumstances (see later in this chapter for further discussion).

But there is a fine level of social differentiation in health risks (the 'fine grain' effect) in that, for example, those with a car and a garden can expect to live longer than those with only a car (Macintyre *et al.*, 1998). This illustrates the phenomena that, at every level of the social hierarchy, including the very highest echelons, there are health differences. This has led health analysts to think about different ways in which hierarchical social location influences our work and social relations, lifestyle and psychological reactions, in ways which are likely to affect health outcomes. The most famous study of this was the British Whitehall Study (Marmot *et al.*, 1978). Although all the people in this study were white-collar workers, there was a huge difference in mortality between the bottom and top grades within the Whitehall hierarchy. The authors concluded that this difference was due not just to more risky lifestyle behaviours (e.g. smoking, eating saturated fats) in the lower grades, but to psychosocial factors to do with work such as lower control over the working environment, greater stress and lower self-worth.

The relationship between wealth and health is discussed further in Chapter 5. The influences of ethnicity, age and gender on health are now highlighted as three specific examples of how social factors can influence health and healthcare.

Ethnicity and health

Global migration trends mean healthcare providers increasingly encounter patients who vary significantly in terms of language, illness-related beliefs and practices and healthcare expectations. Culture influences morbidity and mortality across a wide range of disease areas, and ethnic minorities in all countries tend to have lower socioeconomic status and receive a lower quality of healthcare than non-minorities, even when access-related factors are taken into account. For example, in the UK, cardiovascular disease and cardiovascular risk factors vary dramatically by ethnic group (see 'What's the evidence?' below).

What's the evidence?

Cardiovascular disease, risk factors, and ethnic group

Relative to white European populations, generally people of African origin, Caribbeans and West Africans are less susceptible to coronary heart disease (CHD). On the other hand, South Asian Indians from the Indian subcontinent and from East Africa have a much higher incidence of CHD. Of note is that the poorest ethnic groups in the UK, particularly Pakistanis and Bangladeshis, have the highest mortality rates from CHD. With respect to gender, the patterns for cardiovascular morbidity and mortality in men and women differ, with Bangladeshi and Pakistani men being most affected whereas in women, the Indian and Irish predominate (Cappuccio, 2004).

Interestingly, while ethnicity is the main factor underpinning these differences across groups, differences to do with culture also contribute to these trends (e.g. smoking rates, poorer access to specialised clinical cardiovascular care, economic disadvantage). Furthermore, ethnic and cultural differences can lead to communication problems and act as barriers to care. Empirical studies have identified three different levels of potential barriers to the use of health services among ethnic minority migrants – patient level (e.g. mastery of the local language), provider level (e.g. provider skills and attitudes) and system level (e.g. the organisation of referral and appointments systems) – which interact with each other (Hawthorne *et al.*, 2003).

As stated above, ethnic minorities in all countries tend to have lower socio-economic status. Health disparities related to socio-economic disadvantage can be alleviated, in part, by creating and maintaining culturally competent healthcare systems that can at least overcome communication barriers that may preclude appropriate diagnosis, treatment and follow-up. Providing culturally competent care has the potential to improve health outcomes, increase the efficiency of clinical and support staff and result in greater client satisfaction with services. Culturally competent care brings together a combination of attitudes, skills and knowledge that allows healthcare providers to better understand and take care of patients whose cultural backgrounds, religious beliefs or gender are different from their own (Helman, 2007). What does this mean in practice?

ACTIVITY 4.3

Firstly, familiarise yourself with information about ethnic and cultural groups in your university, hospital or practice catchment area, e.g. what are normal practices in those groups in relation to death and dying? Look at what is available on the Internet for patients whose first language is not English (e.g. Language Line or translation services). Booking longer appointment times will often facilitate the consultation process with patients from different cultural and language backgrounds. Ask colleagues and friends from ethnic and cultural groups other than your own what is considered polite in terms of, for example, personal space. If in doubt, ask!

Cultural competency is not about segregated healthcare. Rather it is about patients coming to an environment specifically designed to put them at ease and offer care that is attuned to their needs who have a better experience and better health as a result. Instead of presenting a way to limit care, cultural competence provides a way to deliver optimal care.

Age and health

Age and health is presented from a psychological perspective in Chapter 3. Here we briefly discuss age from a sociological perspective.

Improvements in sanitation and healthcare have led to more and more people surviving into very old age and dependency giving cause for concern in post-industrial societies such as the UK. Between 1984 and 2009 the proportion of people older than 65 has increased from 15 to 16 per cent, an increase of 1.7 million people, whilst the proportion of young people (<16 years) decreased from 21 to 19 per cent in the UK (National Statistics Online 2010, **www.statistics.gov.uk/cci/nugget. asp?id=949**).

The general population and the media may refer to an unfavourable dependency ratio (number of non-tax payers to be supported by those paying tax) and hence the burden of an ageing population. The debate in several European countries about increasing the retirement age is a good indication of the interaction between biology (i.e. we live longer and are healthier in old age; see Chapter 3) and the economic need for a workforce as well as the social needs of older people's sense of belonging and feeling valued.

Cultures vary greatly in how they value and treat older people. Whilst discriminating against older people in Western societies is legally unacceptable, there may be subtle attempts to keep them out of certain positions for example, as television presenters. In times of healthcare rationing, they may be deemed too old or too uneconomic to benefit from certain medical treatments which would enhance their quality of life.

Gender and health

Sociologists distinguish between *sex* – the biological given – and *gender* – the socially ascribed role. The distinction between sex and gender is fundamental, since many differences between males and females are not biological in origin. The female's biological ability to bear and nurture children does not mean that she has to stay at home and raise them. Nor does men's inability to bear children mean that they have to perform the role of 'breadwinner', bringing home a wage sufficient for the whole family to thrive. Nevertheless, in many developed countries, men still earn more than women and gender roles are still assigned, women for instance often looking after the family's health and accompanying children and older people to the doctor or hospital. Because of this, women are more likely to use preventive services; they may be more in tune with their bodies and more educated about health issues.

In developed countries, women outlive men by four to five years. Thus a larger proportion of the population will be female the older one gets, women are more likely to be in a position of poverty than men and they appear to suffer more ill health during their lives, visiting the doctor more often and suffering more depression. This is not true of undeveloped countries where women are more at risk of dying during or after childbirth. It may be that female hormones protect women from some of the diseases that kill men earlier in life. For example, one in five men dies of heart disease compared with one in seven women but women lose this advantage once they pass the menopause. Also women's increasing involvement in the labour force may be affecting their vulnerability to heart disease. It may be that the pressure of living dual roles – women still do most of the childcare and housework – adversely affects their health. This may be especially true as most societies are patriarchal and women have to live and progress in a male-dominated hierarchy. But we should not ignore the sexism that surrounds attitudes to heart disease; there is plenty of evidence, for example, that women with symptoms receive poorer care because it is assumed that heart disease is only common in men. Because women live longer than men, they suffer more of the chronic diseases of old age such as cancer and heart disease but they are also more prone to some diseases such as osteoporosis.

ACTIVITY 4.4

Go to the main websites concerned with stroke in the UK, such as the British Heart Foundation (**www.bhf.org.uk**).
What are the differences in the incidence of different kinds of stroke in men and women, and in different ages and ethnic groups?
What explanations are there for these differences?

> For example, is it connected to the way that men and women present symptoms?
> Are people from different ethnic groups more stoical or could they be alienated by the healthcare system?
> How many of these groups die as a result of a stroke and why are there these variations in age, gender and ethnic group?

Medical sociology

The Sociology of Health and Illness or Medical Sociology, as it is sometimes called, applies the methods and theories of sociology to the field of health. Health and illness are part of the social world (of people), as is the doctor or the health visitor. Medical sociology studies people's interactions with those engaged in medical occupations, as well as the way people make sense of illness.

Within medical sociology are many sub-disciplines concerned with specific aspects of health and illness such as human reproduction, mental health, lay and professional behaviour, and health promotion. For example, despite inherent risks, pregnancy and childbirth used to be seen as normal and natural processes but now are medically managed (van Teijlingen *et al.*, 2004). The potential of childbirth to go wrong resulting in the death of mother and baby, though rare in developed countries, has resulted in more than 98 per cent of babies in the UK being delivered in hospitals. This is referred to as *medicalisation*, the process whereby more and more areas of human behaviour come to be defined as medical problems often with pharmaceutical or medical solutions (see also Chapter 1, Activity 1.2). For example, medicalisation has lead to problematic patterns of alcohol, gambling and even sex to be reclassified as 'addictions' to be medically managed and children who cannot sit still and concentrate for long have been labelled 'hyperactive' and their behaviour changed by medication.

Sociology also studies the behaviour and interactions of healthcare professionals in their work setting. This could be the study of GPs interacting with fellow doctors, receptionists, and practice nurses, or the interaction between doctors and patients in a consultation. Lingard and colleagues, for example, studied communication between nurses and surgeons during 128 hours of observing 35 different procedures in the operating room and categorised recurrent patterns of communication. They then used their findings to draw links between interpersonal tensions, the use of language and the occurrence of errors in the operating room (Lingard *et al.*, 2004).

The macro level

At the *macro* level, medical sociologists study the patterns of disease found in societies and their possible causes. For example, 11.4 million working days were lost in 2008–09 in Britain as a result of 'stress'. Defined as 'the adverse reaction people have to excessive pressure or other types of demand placed on them' (UK Government Health & Safety Executive), stress is a relatively modern disease, unknown in wartime Britain, which nevertheless affects one in six of those in work, and has individual (e.g. poorer physical and mental health) and social consequences (work days lost, loss of productivity) and consequences in terms of healthcare usage (a significant proportion of patient GP visits are about work-related conditions). Stress at work can lead to lowered mental well-being, physical ill health and health-damaging behaviours (e.g. smoking, bad diet). Sociological studies have shown that factors such as lack of power and control in the workplace, job security, low pay, chequered work security (e.g. changing job frequently, multiple redundancies) are associated with work-related stress.

Many sociological theories have been developed and applied to explore the relationship between work, stress and ill health. Most of these are beyond the remit of this book but it is of interest that work stress has been medicalised (see above): people suffering from work stress (often poorly defined) are encouraged to see themselves as ill, in need of the ministrations of experts (e.g. doctors, stress management counsellors, alternative therapists, self-help materials) who are considered to know much more about their problems than they do. However, research suggests that organisational solutions which address the causes of stress such as workload, role clarity and organisational support (primary prevention) are more effective than those targeted at individual coping (secondary prevention) or counselling (tertiary prevention: see Chapters 5 and 6 for further discussion of health prevention and occupational medicine).

The micro level

At the *micro* level, medical sociologists study the ways that people interpret their symptoms, making sense of illness episodes and their interactions with health professionals. The interpretation of symptoms varies from culture to culture and by gender and age. For example in Latin America, Type II diabetes is often considered to be caused by 'gusto', or shock, whereas in the UK most lay people believe diabetes is linked to diet and obesity. In Africa, hallucinations are often interpreted as due to witchcraft, while in the developed world, they are more likely to be seen as a symptom of psychosis. A mother may seek medical help for a symptom experienced by her child or an elderly relative, which she would ignore in herself because she believes it has greater significance in children (see Chapters 3 and 4 also). The doctor whom she consults may agree and prescribe appropriate treatment or may act in a way the mother does not expect such as dismissing her as 'worrying unnecessarily'.

Interaction between patients and doctors has been studied at this level in an attempt to better understand the doctor–patient relationship. Some research has concentrated on differences in power and 'dominance' between patients and doctors (see Chapter 1). Others have examined more closely the process of becoming a patient and the way that doctors and patients speak to each other and negotiate this shared definition of the situation (McKinstry, 1992; Szasz and Hollander, 1956). Patients recount their experiences in such a way as to convince the doctor of their meaning and significance, often telling a story in the process.

Interestingly, studies have found that verbal communication contributes very little to the impact of the doctor's message, tone of voice contributes quite a lot, but patients are most influenced by non-verbal behaviour (body language). In short, it seems that it is not so much what you say as much as how you say it! Studies into doctor–patient communication have informed the content of clinical communication (often called communication skills) teaching in UK medical schools.

ACTIVITY 4.5

Your clinical communication teaching will involve learning not just what to say to a patient (e.g. when to use open questions rather than closed questions) but also how to say it (e.g. facing the patient, using eye contact, using an encouraging and/or empathic tone of voice). In your next clinical communication session, consciously try to use different tones of voice, or different body language. Reflect on the impact these changes had on the consultation. For example, if you purposively used a calm tone of voice, did your 'patient' seem reassured?

Other studies show that patients often come out of a consultation without having said or done what they had planned for a number of reasons. These include feeling it was not appropriate, feeling too rushed (not wholly unsurprising when the time available for a general practice consultation is usually less than eight minutes), feeling the doctor 'blocked' their attempts to speak about emotive issues, and fearing the doctor's reaction to their experience. Research shows that these patient–doctor communication difficulties are exacerbated when the patient is not of the same culture or gender as the doctor, or speaks a different language (Hawthorne *et al.*, 2003).

As a medical student, you will be trained in problem-solving and active intervention in patients' health complaints. Taking a full, holistic history – not just the history of the presenting problem – is essential in trying to tease out to what extent patients' problems have a social, rather than, or in addition to, a medical origin. However, when social issues (e.g. work-related stress, poor living conditions) are clearly contributing to presentation, response to treatment, etc. dilemmas may arise within the consultation. Patients generally expect more than health or lifestyle advice or a listening ear. In turn, doctors often want to help by treating symptoms, even where it is clear to both parties that this is not really tackling the crux of the problem.

Medical sociology is also relevant to health promotion, discussed in detail in Chapter 6. It is worth mentioning here that promoting healthy behaviour and preventing ill health is only possible if we understand the ways different groups in society, men and women, rich and poor, young and old operate. Sociology provides health promotion practitioners with an analysis of the different groups in society. Thus, the analysis of beliefs regarding tobacco might differ between men and women, smokers and non-smokers, between old and young people, between people with a lower and higher socio-economic background, and between people with higher and lower education. The greater our knowledge of each groups' beliefs, attitudes, prejudices, interests and concerns is, the better the particular health promotion activity can be targeted to a specific group. For example, there is evidence that better-off people generally respond better to health campaigns: people from higher social classes stopped smoking long before the recent legislation banning smoking in public places in the UK. Sociology may help identify ways to effectively encourage smoking cessation in people from lower social classes.

Illness versus disease

Sociologists often distinguish between illness and disease. *Illness* is seen as what people experience when they are unwell, how they interpret or define those symptoms and what actions they take in response to them. There are cultural variations in what are defined as symptoms, in levels of tolerance for pain and in perceptions of appropriate responses. For example, labour pain is part of childbirth, but in some cultures, such as in the UK, it is not accepted and therefore various means are used to alleviate it (e.g. entonox, pethidine, epidural, TENS machines). In some other cultures, labour pain is not only expected but also accepted, and consequently nothing or little is done to relieve it (van Teijlingen *et al.*, 2004).

Often people only seek medical help when symptoms interfere with work or daily life, when they can no longer explain them or when prompted to do so by someone close to them (Zola, 1973). *Disease* is seen as more objective, referring to the signs which a doctor detects and interprets, and the actions which he or she suggests are appropriate responses, e.g. medication or bed rest. In Western societies, doctors often act as gate keepers, issuing or withholding sick notes or prescriptions and thereby legitimising illness. Those whose illness is accepted as genuine are allowed to adopt the *sick role*, a term introduced by Talcott Parsons in the 1950s to describe the privileges and obligations which accompany illness. For example, patients are not held responsible for their illness which is seen as temporary and because of it they are relieved of any responsibility for work and normal activities (Table 4.1). They are however obliged to get well as soon as possible and to seek competent medical help if appropriate.

Table 4.1 Overview of the sick role

Sick role patient	Healthcare professional role
The sick role exempts ill people from their daily responsibilities.	Professional must be objective and not judge patients morally.
Patient is not responsible for being ill, she is regarded as unable to get better without the help of a professional.	Professional must not act out of self-interest or greed but put patient's interests first. He/she must obey a professional code of practice.
Patient must seek help from a healthcare professional.	Professional must have and maintain the necessary knowledge and skills to treat patients.
Patient is under a social obligation to get better as soon as possible to be able to take up social responsibilities again.	Professional has right to examine patient intimately, prescribe treatment and has wide autonomy in medical practice.

ACTIVITY 4.6

Make a list of the expectations that we have of the health professionals who treat patients in terms of their behaviour and the questions they can and cannot ask. What happens when a health professional asks what are seen as inappropriate questions?

What are the rights and obligations of a doctor when working with ill people? Rights and obligations refer to what they are allowed or expected to do in order to treat patients. Think of an example of a mismatch between the patient's expectations and the professional's rights and obligations.

Some illnesses do not justify people claiming all the rights of the sick role, e.g. minor ailments such as colds and stomach upsets may be self-treated and should not require time off work. In such circumstances, an inappropriate adoption of the sick role may be met with a lack of sympathy from family and others such as work colleagues (you will have heard people who have taken time off sick being described as 'swinging the lead', or 'pushing it'). Sometimes people are held responsible for their health condition (e.g. lung cancer or HIV) and because they violate the sick role by being personally responsible (due to having smoked or an involvement in risky sexual behaviour), they may be ostracised. Likewise, people who do not comply or cooperate with treatment plans may be criticised for failing to fulfil their duties to get better. The sick role is socially constructed and sanctioned; people with chronic obstructive lung disease (COPD) often say they wish their disabilities were more evident as they feel they are negatively judged for having a disabled parking permit but looking healthy enough through the eyes of the naïve observer. Those whose diseases are medically unexplained such as chronic fatigue syndrome can feel similarly that they do not have a legitimate claim to the sick role and are not taken seriously as a result.

Parsons's model of the sick role has been criticised for being too simplistic and not taking into account factors such as the growing emphasis on patient empowerment and participation in decision-making. Furthermore, being sick does not automatically lead to becoming a patient as people often rely on lay opinions and advice from others rather than seeking a professional consultation. In other circumstances, such as pregnancy being a patient does not always involve being sick. However, it is a useful lens for thinking about how an individual is managing health and illness, particularly in relation to secondary gains. By secondary gains, we mean the additional benefits that people get from being classed as 'sick'. Such factors include care, sympathy, and concern from family and friends; financial allowances associated with disability; using an apparently disabling illness as an explanation for one's failures; affording the means of avoiding work; restoring status or domination in the family; and achieving revenge for bad treatment or bad pay by an employer or an insurance company. This is a fascinating and controversial topic, particularly in societies with financial systems (such as health insurance and social benefits), which provide support for individuals who are ill and who cannot work.

Often there is a mismatch between patients' and medical professionals' perceptions of illness and disease, possibly due to reliance on different models of health and illness. Doctors are generally seen as relying on the medical model of causation and treatment, and patients a more social one. The doctor's background includes his/her education and experience, continuous updating from peer-reviewed journals and evidence-based medicine (EBM) sources (see Chapter 7 for further discussion of EBM) and other health professionals. The patient's referents may be friends and family members, the media and the Internet. As a result, doctors and patients may have different perceptions of the cause of the condition and the appropriate treatment.

This mismatch is perhaps most apparent with respect to both mental illness and disability, which has resulted in a radical critique of mainstream attitudes. The disability lobby argues that it is inappropriate to use the medical model when dealing with disability when there is often no treatment and no expectation of a return to 'normal' life and responsibilities. A change in social and political attitudes towards disability and disabled living is demanded, rather than concentrating on disabled people's limits and experiences. See Table 4.2 for a comparison of the difference between the medical and social models of disability. Disability is discussed in more depth in Chapter 8. The politicisation of disability has resulted in many changes to the infrastructure of society such as disabled ramps, parking spaces, rights to job interviews, etc., which have increased the awareness if not the support of the able-bodied population.

Table 4.2 Models of disability

Medical	*Social*
Individual/ personal cause e.g. accident resulting from inebriation. Underlying pathology e.g. morbid obesity. Individual level intervention e.g. health professionals advise individually. Individual change/adjustment e.g. change in behaviour.	Societal cause e.g. low wages. Conditions relating to environment e.g. damp housing. Social/political action needed e.g. facilities for disabled. Societal attitude change e.g. use of politically correct language.

Case study

Bill is working class, a baker by trade but he now works as a payroll administrator for the same company where he worked first as an apprentice, and then as a master baker. He enjoys the social aspect of work; he goes for a pint with his colleagues on payday, the members of his curling team are all work colleagues. Although the UK smoking ban means smoking in pubs is no longer allowed, Bill and his mates make daily use of the smoking shelter in the workplace car park. Their attitude is that the smoking ban is an infringement of their individual human rights, and they are determined to keep smoking on principle! Susan thinks this is nonsense and would really like Bill to quit but he is torn between keeping his family happy and being 'one of the boys'.

How could the smoking behaviour of Bill and his workmates be considered in terms of group/community norms? Consider how Bill's membership of different groups (his workmates, his family) seems to be the cause of interpersonal conflict?

Also, redundancies are threatened at work due to the recession. Bill is anxious about this – the family could not manage without his income. He finds having a cigarette calms him down, gives him a break from worrying about his job.

If Bill is made redundant and cannot find alternative employment, the family's income will drop significantly. What could be the impact of this in terms of the 'health gradient'?

Chapter summary

This chapter has discussed a number of key concepts in sociology and their application in medical sociology. It has shown how medical sociological perspectives are relevant to our understanding of health and illness and the practice of medicine. It has demonstrated the possibility of referring to competing explanations when examining important social differences such as social class, and wealth, and mortality or gender roles and morbidity. The influence of gender, age and ethnicity on health has been highlighted as particular examples. It has shown that relationships such as those between doctor and patient or mother and child are subject to social forces that change over time and between societies.

GOING FURTHER

Alder, B, Abraham, C, van Teijlingen, E and Porter, M (eds) (2009) *Psychology and Sociology: Applied to Medicine*, 3rd edition. Edinburgh: Churchill Livingstone/ Elsevier.
An illustrated colour text covering all aspects of the lifespan as well as health promotion, society and health and how health services work, to name but a few.

chapter 5

Populations, Health and Disease

Karen Foster, Cairns Smith and
Edwin van Teijlingen

Achieving your medical degree

This chapter will help you to meet the following requirements of *Tomorrow's Doctors* (2009).

11 Apply to medical practice the principles, method and knowledge of population health and the improvement of health and healthcare.

   (a) Discuss basic principles of health improvement, including the wider determinants of health, health inequalities, health risks and disease surveillance.
   (b) Assess how health behaviours/outcomes are affected by diversity of the patient population.
   (c) Describe measurement methods relevant to improvement of clinical effectiveness and care.
   (d) Discuss the principles underlying the development of health and health service policy, including issues relating to health economics and equity, and clinical guidelines.
   (f) Evaluate and apply epidemiological data in managing healthcare for the individual and the community.
   (h) Discuss the role of nutrition in health.
   (j) Discuss from a global perspective the determinants of health and disease and variations in healthcare delivery and medical practice.

Chapter overview

After reading this chapter, you will be able to demonstrate an understanding of the following:

- Population influences on health, including differences in healthcare development, delivery and policy across different countries, and even regions.
- Approaches to measuring and addressing population influences on health.
- The relevance and practice of epidemiolog.
- Some of the factors which influence how disease is treated.

Introduction

Public health is concerned with the health of a whole population, less about individual patients. Public health attempts, through scientific enquiry, to discover the best ways of eliminating or preventing disease on a population scale, rather than treating individual cases. This approach is essential as many of the factors that influence health operate at the level of society and are, to an extent, out of the control of individuals (e.g. inequality, poverty, education). While most medical disciplines cover aspects of prevention and health promotion, most of their work is curative and caring. Public health has a slightly different perspective on health and well-being, one which is more based on the notion of positive health, to improve lives through the prevention and treatment of disease, prolonging life and promoting health through the organised efforts of society. This involves mobilising individuals, groups and the body of societal or governmental machinery in order to put the strategies into action for the benefit of the public's health. This means public health is also concerned with designing health services, evaluating their effectiveness, and making decisions about the allocation of resources. Figure 5.1 shows the main elements of public health.

The 10 Essential Elements of Public Health

Public Health has identified the following 10 essential elements that define public health practice:

1.	**Monitor health status** to identify community health problems
2.	**Diagnose and investigate** health problems and health hazards in the community
3.	**Inform, educate, and empower** people about health issues
4.	**Mobilize community partnerships** to identify and solve health problems
5.	**Develop policies and plans** that support individual and community health efforts
6.	**Enforce laws and regulations** that protect health and ensure safety
7.	**Link people to needed personal health service** and assure the provision of health care when otherwise unavailable
8.	**Assure a competent workforce** for public health and personal health care
9.	**Evaluate effectiveness,** accessibility and quality of personal and population based services
10.	**Research for new insights** and innovative solutions to health problems

Figure 5.1 The 10 essential elements of public health.

Source: Adapted from **www.fph.org.uk/what_is_public_health**.

The World Health Organization's (WHO's) (1946) definition of health as 'a state of complete physical, mental, and social well-being, and not merely the absence of disease or infirmity' is useful to recall here as this definition is also based on the notion of positive health. Examples of public health achievements in the UK include clean air and water, enhanced nutrition and mass immunisation, all of which have improved health outcomes for millions of people.

This example illustrates how modern public health is usually concerned with addressing determinants of health across a population, rather than advocating for individual behaviour change. Modern public health is called *population health*. Population health seeks to address health inequalities by advocating for population-based policies that improve health in an equitable manner.

Before we can decide how we could or should go about improving the health of a population we need to establish what the problems are and whose health status we are aiming to improve, and thereafter we need to be able to measure whether we have improved health, or not.

Global patterns of health and healthcare

In terms of identifying the problem(s), the WHO provides estimates of those diseases that contribute most to the death rate worldwide (Table 5.1). Top of the list is heart disease; nearly one in eight of the global population dies of ischaemic heart disease. Globally, 60 per cent of deaths relate to non-communicable conditions, 30 per cent is due to communicable, reproductive or nutritional conditions and 10 per cent is caused by injuries.

Table 5.1 Leading causes of death worldwide per year, as established by the WHO

Disease or injury	Deaths (millions)	Total deaths %
1. Ischaemic heart disease	7.2	12.2
2. Cerebrovascular disease	5.7	9.7
3. Lower respiratory infections	4.2	7.1
4. COPD	3.0	5.1
5. Diarrhoeal diseases	2.2	3.7
6. HIV/AIDS	2.0	3.5
7. Tuberculosis	1.5	2.5
8. Trachea, bronchus, lung cancers	1.3	2.3
9. Road traffic accidents	1.3	2.2
10. Prematurity and low birth weight	1.2	2.0
11. Neonatal infections+	1.1	1.9
12. Diabetes mellitus	1.1	1.9
13. Hypertensive heart disease	1.0	1.7
14. Malaria	0.9	1.5
15. Birth asphyxia and birth trauma	0.9	1.5
16. Self-inflicted injuries*	0.8	1.4

17. Stomach cancer	0.8	1.4
18. Cirrhosis of the liver	0.8	1.3
19. Nephritis and nephrosis	0.7	1.3
20. Colon and rectum cancers	0.6	1.1

Source: Adapted from WHO (2008a).

+ This category also includes other non-infectious causes arising in the perinatal period, apart from prematurity, low birth weight, birth trauma and asphyxia. These non-infectious causes are responsible for about 20 per cent of deaths shown in this category.

* Self-inflicted injuries resulting in death can also be referred to as suicides.

However, the burden of disease is not the same across the globe, disease patterns vary considerably both between and within countries. For example, in low-income countries the top three killer diseases are lower respiratory infections, coronary heart disease and diarrhoeal diseases, whilst in the high-income countries, the top three causes of death are coronary heart disease, stroke and other cerebrovascular diseases, followed by trachea, bronchus and lung cancers. Neither are patterns of disease static: improved standards of living and medical advances change the patterns of disease. For example, some infectious diseases have been virtually eradicated, such as measles, but others have emerged, for example HIV/AIDS. Thus, population health goals and strategies differ by place and time.

As well as burden of disease, population health also focusses on health risks, the risks responsible for mortality – understanding these is key to preventing disease and injury. The leading global risks for mortality in the world are high blood pressure, tobacco use, high blood glucose, physical inactivity, and overweight and obesity (WHO Global Health Risks, 2009a). This same report identified five leading risk factors are responsible for one quarter of all deaths in the world (childhood underweight (e.g. due to malnutrition), unsafe sex, alcohol use, unsafe water and sanitation, and high blood pressure). Reducing exposure to these risk factors would increase global life expectancy by nearly 5 years. Low-income populations are most affected by risks associated with poverty, such as undernutrition – children being underweight is the biggest risk factor or leading cause of death in low-income countries.

As disease burden and health risks differ across countries, so do population health goals: the focus of public health in a country with inadequate sanitation and with widespread malnutrition is different from those in a country with clean water and food available to all. Population health goals also differ across areas within the same country; for example, in the UK, addressing health inequalities in terms of differing access to services between urban and rural areas, and between wealthy and poorer urban areas, is a current priority.

ACTIVITY 5.1 WHY DO DISEASE PATTERNS DIFFER BETWEEN HIGH- AND LOW-INCOME COUNTRIES?

Search for the report on Global Health Risks, under Health Statistics on the WHO website (**www.who.int/healthinfo/global_burden_disease/global_health_risks/en/index.html**).

What are the main differences in disease patterns between high- and low-income countries? How do different risk factors contribute to specific diseases? Thinking beyond the data presented in this report, consider the influence of social and environmental factors such as societal norms, or the way healthcare systems are organised, or natural disasters, on disease patterns and health risks?

It is not just the burden of disease which differs across countries: healthcare systems are organised very differently in different countries. The UK has a comprehensive health service, funded through taxation, with healthcare free at the point of care open to everybody living in the country, with no payment upfront for public healthcare. Many other countries have a mixed economy of healthcare in which some core services are government-funded and other services are accessed through a market-based healthcare system where people have to pay for certain treatments or basic healthcare. In countries such as the USA, poor people may find it very hard to afford or get access to good healthcare. Similarly, in developing countries like Nepal or Bangladesh, certain services are freely available to the population, but patients need to pay, for example, for medications, laboratory investigations, etc. A third way of organising health involves a mixed economy between private and government health insurance schemes, where people have to subscribe to a scheme which will reimburse hospitals, doctors, physiotherapists and midwives for services offered to an insured patient. Such national health insurance schemes can be found in countries such as Germany and the Netherlands.

Furthermore, while most countries have their own government public health agencies (e.g. England has the Department of Health [DH]) in the developing world, many public health infrastructures are still forming and there may not be enough trained health workers or monetary resources to provide even a basic level of medical care and disease prevention. As a result, a large majority of disease and mortality in the developing world results from, and contributes to, extreme poverty.

In short, health problems and health services differ across the world and the focus and capacity of population health efforts is therefore different across countries. Key problems might be mental health in rural Scotland, the transmission of HIV/AIDS in Africa or obesity in children in Central America. The target population (those whose health status we are aiming to improve) might be unemployed men, sex workers or mothers and these target groups may change over time as disease patterns change.

Identifying the problem: the role of epidemiology

Health problems need to be defined and measured so population health doctors and policy makers know which problems to address, and whether interventions designed to do so have been effective and efficient. *Epidemiology* is the study of changing patterns of disease with a main aim of improving the health of populations. Essentially, epidemiology compares the event rate of a particular disease across groups (e.g. men and women, different countries, different ethnic groups) to detect differences that provide pointers as to the spread of disease progression (disease surveillance), what might be causing disease, the scope for prevention and the identification of high risk priority groups within society who may benefit from an intervention. Epidemiology is the cornerstone of population health research, central to the health of society, to the identification of causes of disease, and to their management and prevention.

Epidemiology has had an impact on many areas of medicine, from discovering the relationship between tobacco smoking and lung cancer to the origin and spread of new epidemics. However, it is often poorly understood, possibly because it involves clinical trials and statistics (see Chapter 7 for more discussion of the research methods used in epidemiology). Some understanding of a few basic concepts (prevalence, incidence and relative risk) and how epidemiology can be used might help demystify this subject.

The distribution of health-related states or events can be described in terms of time, place and person. When considering the spread of disease in a population we need to make a distinction between the 'prevalence' of a disease and the 'incidence'.

Prevalence is the number of people in a population with a specific disease at a single point of time (point prevalence) or in a defined period of time (period prevalence). The prevalence of asthma in children in Britain was recently (Burr *et al.*, 2006) estimated at one in 11 or 9 per cent, one of the highest rates in the world.

The *incidence* is the number of new cases of disease in a population in a specified period of time. For example, the incidence of asthma in children (number of new cases per year) is thought to have levelled off in recent years following a period of rising numbers of children developing the illness. Pollution, burger eating, allergens and failure to be breastfed have all been examined as possible reasons for the worldwide increase in incidence of asthma in children. At the same time we need to bear in mind that part of the increased incidence of many diseases is increased knowledge/evidence, and hence better recognition and diagnosis.

Another basic epidemiological concept is *relative risk (RR)* – the risk of an event (or of developing a disease) relative to exposure (e.g. smokers have a higher relative risk of developing lung cancer than non-smokers).

ACTIVITY 5.2

What would the characteristics be of a disease with a high incidence but low prevalence?

Can you think of such a disease?

The relationship between prevalence and incidence is affected by the duration of the disease. You have to bear in mind that prevalence can only change if individuals get better or die. Winter flu in the UK has, in a short period over the winter months, a high incidence and prevalence with hundreds of thousands of people affected for a short period of time, most getting better rapidly within weeks. Motor neurone disease (amyotrophic lateral sclerosis [ALS]), a degenerative neurological disorder, has a low prevalence in the UK population of about 7 per 100,000 but compared to the prevalence rate, a relatively high incidence rate of 2 per 100,000. The reason that the prevalence rate does not change much from year to year is that roughly the same number of people die of the disease who get diagnosed in a year.

The importance of epidemiology in day-to-day medical practice is best illustrated with an example (see 'What's the evidence?' below), which demonstrates the distribution of COPD in terms of time (increasing prevalence to 2020), place (urban/rural, North of England, European distribution) and person (gender, age), and the determinants of COPD (smoking, social inequalities, exposure to occupational vapours, gas, dust and fumes).

What's the evidence?

The epidemiology of COPD

Chronic obstructive pulmonary disease (COPD) is thought to be the fourth most common cause of death worldwide and the WHO anticipates that by 2020 it will have become the third. This likely increase is primarily related to changes in smoking behaviour in the developing world and changes in the population age structures.

In 2004, 27,478 men and women living in the UK died of COPD, the vast majority (more than 90 per cent) of these deaths occurring in those older than 65 years.

Mortality from COPD in England shows a strong urban rural gradient with high mortality rates in the large conurbations in the north of England. There are also striking social inequalities with men aged 20–64 years employed in unskilled manual occupations being 14 times more likely to die from COPD than those in professional occupations.

A systematic review of all population-based studies of COPD from anywhere in the world and published from 1990 to 2004 estimated that the prevalence of COPD in adults above the age of 40 years was 9–10 per cent.

This figure fails to capture variation in age-specific rates and variation in prevalence with a history of past and current smoking in these older generations. In adults under the age of 45 years living in Europe the prevalence of COPD as defined by GOLD stage criteria is about 2.5% for Stage 1 (Mild COPD – mild airflow limitation [FEV1/FVC < 0.70; FEV1 $\rightarrow$ 80% predicted]) and about 1%

> *for stage 2 (Moderate COPD – characterized by worsening airflow limitation [FEV1/FVC < 0.70; 50% " FEV1 < 80% predicted]) or 3 (Severe COPD – characterized by further worsening of airflow limitation [FEV1/FVC < 0.70; 30% " FEV1 < 50% predicted]). This study suggests that the prevalence of disease in young adults in the UK is about average compared to other European countries. In all countries the prevalence of the disease was associated with smoking and exposure to occupational vapours, gas, dust and fumes.*
>
> (Burney and Jarvis, 2006)

The example of COPD illustrates how epidemiological information can be used to

- assist in making a diagnosis of COPD – A man presents with cough, phlegm and shortness of breath. If he is a 65-year old manual worker who has smoked since he was 15, it is very likely that he is suffering from COPD. If he is a 23-year-old office worker who has never smoked the diagnosis of COPD is far less likely.

- assess which services are required for prevention, diagnosis, primary care, secondary care, rehabilitation.

- ensure a high quality of these services (clinical audit, implementation of guidelines, PDSA [*Plan, Do, Study, Act*] cycles – see later in this chapter).

- carry out healthcare needs assessments to provide a rational framework for decisions on prioritisation of COPD healthcare resources.

Epidemiology defines and addresses health problems using a range of research study designs and statistical analyses, discussed further in Chapter 7. Epidemiology also depends on other sources of routinely gathered (rather than research study) data: hospital and clinical activity statistics, general practice data, national surveys, NHS expenditure (e.g. prescription data) and mortality data. These sources of data are invaluable in identifying problems and planning services. Bear in mind, however, that such data is not infallible – for example, not all relevant data may be included in a routine database – and observed differences in data may be due to differences in healthcare practices across countries rather than variations in disease.

Influences on health

Epidemiology tells us that diseases are generally not entities striking randomly in a population: most of the time we can recognise and predict patterns. These patterns can vary by genetic make-up and physiology, geographical area, ethnic background or by social factors. Social factors refer to the cultural, economic and social conditions that shape the health of individuals, communities, and jurisdictions as a whole (see also Dalgren and Whitehead's model in Chapter 1). Social determinants of health include wealth and work (see 'What's the evidence?' below), and the interaction between one's social environmental and individual behaviour (Wilkinson and Marmot, 2003). Health and wealth are entwined: people living in the poorest areas of the UK will, on average, die seven years earlier than people living in richer areas and spend up to 17 more years living with poor health. They have higher rates of mental illness; of harm from alcohol, drugs and smoking; and of childhood emotional and behavioural problems.

The social determinants of health are the conditions in which people are born, grow, live, work and age, including the health system. These circumstances are shaped by the distribution of money, power and resources at global, national and local levels, which are themselves influenced by policy choices. The social determinants of health are mostly responsible for health inequities – the unfair and avoidable differences in health status seen within and between countries.

What's the evidence?

It is important to remember that addressing the social determinants of health at a population level applies to high-income as well as low-income countries. Consider studies of legislative interventions for transport-related injury prevention in developed countries. Systematic reviews of studies of legislative interventions to curb alcohol-impaired driving have found strong evidence for reduction of fatal and non-fatal crash outcomes (Shults *et al.*, 2001). Similarly, traffic calming interventions have been found to deliver reductions in road traffic injuries (Bunn *et al.*, 2003).

The UK government established the National Health Service (NHS) in 1948 with the core aim of improving the health of the population. A draft of health improvement initiatives were set in place over time with a landmark study culminating in the *Black Report* published in 1980 (Townsend and Davidson, 1982). The *Black Report* was the first study to systematically analyse the relationships between wealth, or more accurately social class, and health inequalities in the UK. It came up with four explanations for the differences between social class and health:

(a) cultural (health beliefs, behaviours and expectations – see Chapter 3)

(b) material (resources: income but also housing, working conditions, social environment, education, etc.)

(c) genetic (e.g. gender, ethnicity – see Chapter 4) and

(d) artefact (differences between social classes may not be real but due to how measurements are conducted).

An example of a material resource is food. Many global health inequalities are associated with either a lack of, or an overabundance of, food/nutrition. Many people in developing countries die from diseases which would not normally kill them in developed countries because they are undernourished, which weakens their resistance to other diseases. Conversely, many of the causes of death which are more common in developed countries are linked to obesity, which is in turn due to overnutrition. In fact, obesity kills more people than being underweight. WHO data indicates that being overweight (measured by body mass index [BMI]) is a major risk factor for non-communicable diseases such as cardiovascular diseases, diabetes, musculoskeletal disorders and some cancers. Furthermore, childhood obesity is associated with a higher chance of obesity, premature death and disability in adulthood. But in addition to increased future risks, obese children experience breathing difficulties, increased risk of fractures, hypertension, early markers of cardiovascular disease, insulin resistance and psychological effects (see **www.who.int/mediacentre/factsheets/fs311/en/index.html** for more on nutrition and health inequality).

More recently, the WHO suggested ten key determinants which affect the health status of an individual (see Figure 5.2). Each of these can be influenced by the others. For example, the use of health services can be related to income, especially in countries where the patient has to pay for healthcare out of their own pocket. But the uptake of health services can also be influenced by the physical environment, e.g. patients living in rural areas with poor transport are less likely to use health services when they need them than those living in urban areas.

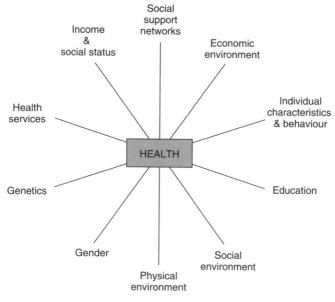

Figure 5.2 Main determinants of health.

Source: Adapted from World Health Organization 2008b.

Research suggests that materialistic (e.g. wealth) and lifestyle/cultural factors are now thought to explain differences across social classes more than the artefact or genetic explanations highlighted in the *Black Report*. This reinforces the message reiterated throughout this book that sensitivity to the background of individual patients is essential to good medical practice, but being aware of the social, cultural and ethnic background of your patients should not lead to stereotyping or attributing everything to such factors.

Much of the health improvement over the past centuries has not been due to individuals changing their health behaviour (eat a bit better or smoke a bit less), but, in keeping with the overarching goals of public health, to changes at a population level; examples include better supply of food, tighter legislation of child labour and quality control of drinking water. The design of population-focussed interventions is discussed in detail in Chapter 6 while evaluation of effectiveness is discussed below.

Clinical effectiveness

NHS Quality Improvement Scotland (NHS QIS) (**www.nhshealthquality.org/nhsqis**) defines clinical effectiveness as the extent to which specific clinical interventions do what they are intended to do; that is, maintain and improve the health of patients securing the greatest possible health gain from the available resources.

Clinical effectiveness is defined by NHS QIS (**www.nhshealthquality.org/nhsqis**) as the right person doing

- the right thing (evidence-based practice)
- in the right way (skills and competence)
- at the right time (providing treatment/services when the patient needs them)
- in the right place (location of treatment/services)
- with the right result (clinical effectiveness/maximising health gain).

Clinical effectiveness involves thinking critically about clinical practice, questioning whether it is having the desired result, and making a change to practice. It is based on evidence of what is effective in order to improve patient care. Clinical effectiveness itself is part of a drive towards evidence-based practice, which is concerned with finding the best available evidence and applying this to a clinical problem in an individual patient, or group of patients.

Individual doctors do not have the time to read all the available clinical research published every week and use the results to decide how to amend their clinical practice. Therefore, there are a number of organisations whose role is to review the available evidence and advise clinicians on best practice. In the UK, the National Institute for Health and Clinical Excellence (NICE) produces clinical guidelines and guidance for the NHS. NICE guidance is designed to promote good health and prevent ill health. NICE guidelines are high quality, the website is updated frequently and it is a very reliable source of clinical information, used not only in the UK but also by clinicians and health services in other countries.

Why is clinical effectiveness important?

Health inequality may arise from variation in clinical practice and in the treatments that patients receive. Before we discuss this, it is worth mentioning that some variation in clinical practice and treatment may be entirely appropriate. An area which has a higher rate of very elderly people will utilise more healthcare resources than an area which has a population of mostly young adults, who tend to be a healthy age group. However, often variation in clinical practice is not appropriate and is an indication of waste or inequity in the NHS. Variation can be seen in many areas of medical practice, including prescribing patterns, rates of certain operations and treatment of conditions such as COPD. Variations which result in overuse or underuse of healthcare resources can be costly and may expose patients to unnecessary risk. Patients may receive treatments which are not very effective or for which there is no evidence, or they may not receive treatments which are evidence-based and effective when they need them.

Inappropriate variation in clinical practice may occur as a result of other factors such as:

- the doctor not being up to date with what is the most effective treatment for a specific condition in a given patient population;
- lack of resources to be able to implement the best practice;
- sufficient overall resources for a specific patient population but allocation of these resources in the wrong way.

Patients have the right to expect the same high standard of care and treatment wherever they access NHS services (healthcare equality). However, we often hear the media and politicians refer to 'postcode prescribing' as an example of inequality based on geography rather than the needs of patients. This can occur as a result of preferences and habits of clinical decision makers, or due to other factors, such as the socioeconomic status of patients.

ACTIVITY 5.4

Type 'postcode prescribing' into your preferred search engine. This will find many different recent articles, from those published in scientific journals, to those published by healthcare and related organisations, to those in national newspapers. Take a few moments to examine some of these articles, to compare and contrast different views of this phenomenon.

Since the NHS started in 1948, the range and complexity of available treatments have grown substantially, as has the public's demand for medical care. The cost of healthcare has also continued to rise. It is therefore essential that the NHS makes the best use of its resources by ensuring that effective interventions are implemented appropriately and ineffective interventions are not used. Thus, clinical effectiveness can be considered a component of public health as it addresses healthcare inequalities, and focusses on improving health and healthcare at a population level.

Quality improvement activities

Clinical effectiveness is made up of a range of quality improvement activities including:

- Evidence, guidelines and standards.
- Quality improvement tools (such as clinical audit, plan do study act (PDSA), root cause analysis, statistical process control and service redesign) to review and improve treatments and services based on
  - the views of patients, service users and staff
  - evidence from incidents, near-misses, clinical risks and risk analysis
  - outcomes from treatments or services
  - measurement of performance to assess whether the team/department/organisation is achieving the desired goals
  - identifying areas of care that need further research.
- Information systems to assess current practice and provide evidence of improvement.
- Assessment of evidence as to whether services/treatments are cost-effective.
- Development and use of systems and structures that promote learning and learning across the organisation.
- Good practice monitoring systems such as the quality outcomes framework (QOF, see later) in general practice.

See NHS Scotland Educational Resources Clinical Governance (**www.clinicalgovernance.scot.nhs.uk**) and Department of Health (**www.dh.gov.uk/en/index.htm**) for more information.

We will discuss some of these activities – evidence, guidelines, standards, and clinical audit – in a little detail.

Evidence, guidelines and standards

As mentioned earlier in this chapter, clinical guidelines are systematically developed statements to assist practitioner and patient decisions about appropriate healthcare for specific clinical circumstances. Guidelines provide recommendations for effective practice in the management of clinical conditions where variations in practice are known to occur and where effective care may not be delivered uniformly. Guideline recommendations might include the use of protocols – predetermined criteria which usually address practical issues (e.g. insulin profusion) or safe practice (e.g. recording swabs, needles and blades in the operating theatre to prevent items of equipment being left inside the patient). Evidence-based medicine is discussed in more detail in Chapter 7.

A clinical standard, in contrast, is something that serves as a basis for comparison to assess quality of care. A clinical standard might specify how patient data should be stored, basic skills and knowledge required by practitioners in relation to patient care and management, service delivery (what, when). Clinical standards focus on providing optimum quality patient care, based on what is known (the evidence) and approved by a recognised and representative body.

In Scotland, NHS Quality Improvement Scotland (NHS QIS) publishes Clinical Standards for a range of services (**www.nhshealthquality.org/nhsqis**). In England, this role is fulfilled by the National Institute for Health and Clinical Excellence (NICE; **www.nice.org.uk**).

ACTIVITY 5.5

NICE and NHS QIS standards are based on best evidence to promote good health and prevent ill health. They have transparent and rigorous procedures for developing and monitoring clinical standards. Go to the NICE (**www.nice.org.uk**) and NHS QIS websites (**www.nhshealthquality.org/nhsqis**) to compare and contract the remit and roles of these two organisations.

The quality and outcomes framework (QOF), introduced in 2004 as part of the General Medical Services Contract with GP practices in the UK rewarding them for how well they care for patients, can be viewed as a set of clinical standards. The QOF contains groups of indicators, against which practices score points according to their level of achievement, in different domains. For example, the 2010/11 QOF clinical indicators for heart failure are as follows:

- *Records*: The practice can produce a register of patients with heart failure.

- *Initial diagnosis*: The percentage of patients with a diagnosis of heart failure (diagnosed after 1 April 2006), which has been confirmed by an echocardiogram or by specialist assessment.

- *Ongoing management*: The percentage of patients with a current diagnosis of heart failure due to left ventricular dysfunction (LVD) who are currently treated with an ACE inhibitor or angiotensin receptor blocker, who can tolerate therapy and for whom there is no contraindication.

- The percentage of patients with a current diagnosis of heart failure due to LVD who are currently treated with an ACE inhibitor or angiotensin receptor blocker, who are additionally treated with a beta-blocker licensed for heart failure, or recorded as intolerant to or having a contraindication to beta-blockers.

The QOF gives an indication of the overall achievement of a practice through a points system. Practices aim to deliver high-quality care across a range of areas, for which they score points.

Quality improvement tools

The main quality improvement tool used by clinicians is clinical audit, a quality improvement process that seeks to improve patient care and outcomes through systematic review of care against explicit criteria and the implementation of change. Clinical audit is an ongoing cycle of continuous improvement and is often represented as an audit cycle or spiral (see Figure 5.3).

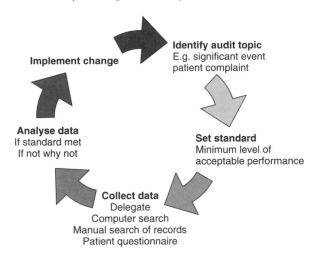

Figure 5.3 The clinical audit cycle.

Source: **www.clinical-audit.org.uk**

Clinical audit is used to compare current practice with evidence of good practice. It can be used to make changes that improve the delivery of care. It can:

- provide evidence of current practice against national guidelines or standards;

- provide information about the structures, the processes or outcomes of a healthcare service;

- assess how closely local practice resembles recommended practice; and

- provide evidence about the quality of care in a service.

Clinical audit is a standard part of the role of a doctor. General practices and hospital-based specialties continually review practice to ensure their patients are receiving good quality care. You may be able to gain experience of audit when on rotation and will certainly be involved in audit when you are a Foundation doctor.

Clinical audit is discussed further in Chapter 7, where the difference between audit and research is described.

Planning health services and healthcare decision-making

Clinical effectiveness and quality improvement tools focus on providing the best healthcare now. Population health is also concerned with planning health services to ensure we have the right type of health services available in the future. Some of the planning is for today, should a major public health disaster happen (e.g. a swine flu epidemic break out) but planners also think ten years ahead (e.g. what hospital facilities will be needed in the next decade? – designing the hospital, raising the funding, getting planning permission, clearing the building site, building the actual building, adding all the latest technology in the wards and theatres can easily take 6 to 8 years). Planners also need to take into consideration the key demands on a healthcare budget.

There are four main factors which influence healthcare planning:

(1) Advances in science and technology
For example, penicillin was discovered by accident in 1928 and started being manufactured in the early 1940s. There are now (2011) twelve categories of antibiotic in the British National Formulary as well as antifungals, antivirals, antiprotozoals and anthelmintics and a major concern is the development of resistance to available treatments caused by overuse of antibiotic therapy.

(2) Changes in the population
The population of the UK is ageing, with the fastest population increase being in those aged 85 years and older. Alemayehu and Warner (2004) showed that nearly one-third of per capita lifetime healthcare expenditure is incurred during middle age, and nearly half during the senior years. For people surviving to age 85, more than one-third of their lifetime expenditures will accrue in their remaining years. Our increasingly elderly population will therefore have a huge impact on healthcare resources. However, bear in mind that age is not the only variable here: most money on healthcare is spent in the last year of life whether people die at age 3, 33 or 93. (Lubitz and Riley, 1993).

(3) Changes in the way care is delivered
Increasingly healthcare is being delivered in the community rather than in hospitals, with shorter lengths of stay for those who are admitted to hospital. Patients are being

encouraged to take more responsibility for their health with self-care and self-management of chronic conditions. Technology advances have revolutionised the way healthcare is delivered including computerisation, telemedicine, keyhole surgery and use of robotics in surgery.

(4) Changes in patients' expectations of healthcare and health services
In the early days of the NHS, patients looked to healthcare professionals to treat their injuries and infections, deliver their babies safely and look after the chronic sick. The elderly were usually looked after by their extended family. There was some health promotion activity but a certain level of maternal and child mortality was accepted and almost every death occurred at home. In the twenty-first century, patients expect health promotion services (weight management, smoking cessation, contraceptive services), prevention initiatives (immunisation, screening programmes, travel advice), management of acute and chronic illness 24/7, cosmetic surgery, fertility treatment, gender realignment and treatment of addiction all from the NHS budget. Very few people die in their own home and indeed death is very often seen as a medical failure.

A major mechanism for planning NHS service provision is through the assessment of the healthcare needs of the population. Health needs assessment is a systematic method for reviewing the health issues facing a population, leading to agreed priorities and resource allocation that will improve health and reduce inequalities. It depends on data on the following:

- Incidence and prevalence (how many people in the community need a particular healthcare intervention);

- Effectiveness (does healthcare intervention produce benefits and at what cost);

- Current service provision (in order to know how services need to be changed).

Need is different from both the 'demand for' and the 'supply of' healthcare. 'Demand' is what services people wish to use in a free healthcare system (or are willing to pay for in a private healthcare system such as in the USA) whilst 'supply' is what is actually provided. Need, demand and supply may or may not overlap. Mismatches between need, supply and demand are commonly seen within the NHS. For example, there is a high demand for infertility services (e.g. in vitro fertilisation [IVF]), which is not met (supplied) currently by the NHS (the need is met for those who can afford treatment in the private sector). Alternatively, there is a high demand and supply of GP services for 'coughs and colds' without any real healthcare need ('coughs and colds' are self-limiting and rarely serious). See Bandolier **www.medicine.ox.ac.uk/bandolier** for more information.

Health economics can help to inform healthcare planning and decision-making by structured evaluations which make explicit the costs and benefits of health interventions. This involves a 'trade-off' between the pros and cons of one intervention versus another: we utilise a resource in one way, we have given up the opportunity of spending it in another beneficial manner. Available resources should therefore be used to provide only those types of healthcare that have been shown to be effective in robust analyses. In addition, these resources must be allocated equitably to those who need them, regardless of, for example, social, ethnic or cultural status.

Health economists utilise techniques to attempt to obtain maximum value for money by ensuring not just the clinical effectiveness (see earlier), but also the cost-effectiveness of healthcare interventions. Economists look at costs that are far wider than just financial costs and include the wider concept of resource consumption, irrespective of whether such resources incur a financial price tag. For example, the time spent by patients and their families in a hospital waiting room represents a real cost, which must be included in the evaluation, even though this incurs no financial cost.

There are four main economic evaluations of healthcare:

- Cost-minimisation analysis is used in situations in which the health benefits of healthcare treatments have been shown to be identical and the cheapest way to deliver this outcome is sought.

- Cost-effectiveness analysis is defined as the ratio of the net change in healthcare costs to the net change in health outcomes. It answers the question – how much more does it cost to achieve an additional unit of benefit?

- Cost-utility analysis measures the effect of an intervention on mortality or morbidity, i.e. quantity or quality of life. A quality-adjusted life year (QALY) measures the number of additional life years obtained from a health intervention, weighted by the quality of life experienced in each year.

- Cost-benefit analysis measures both costs and benefits solely in financial terms. An intervention may then be adopted if the financial price assigned to the benefits is greater than that of the costs.

Economists are also concerned with efficiency, which measures how well resources are used to achieve a desired outcome.

It might seem that healthcare needs assessment should be straightforward, based on a combination of the evidence-based and economic planning/evaluations. However, interested parties (such as professional groups, politicians, managers and the public) have demands, wishes and perspectives. These tend to be based in moral values and personal preferences (e.g. wishing local rather than centralised healthcare delivery) rather than hard-nosed rational decision-making. Broader community issues such as transport, leisure activities and pollution (as well as access to health services) also impact on health. Furthermore, regardless of which government is in power and how much of the overall gross domestic product (GDP) is spent on health, the demand for healthcare will always outstrip the available resources in a healthcare system funded through taxation. Finally, undertaking healthcare needs assessments is often difficult due to inherent uncertainties in attempting to quantify healthcare services, because of:

- inadequate information on the incidence/prevalence of diseases/illnesses,

- inadequate data on effectiveness (and cost-effectiveness),

- lack of agreement on the 'threshold levels' for intervention,

- complex and ill-defined patient pathways into and through the NHS system,

- political and media pressures around the allocation of limited resources,

- competing concerns in attempting to provide healthcare that is both: effective, efficient, equitable, affordable, accessible and appropriate.

ACTIVITY 5.6

If you were a healthcare planner in your home town (or village) and you were given substantial extra funding what type of healthcare (drug, intervention, prevention, patient group, locality, etc.) would you spend it on? How would you know your decision would be the best use of the extra resources?

In reality, healthcare policy, decision-making and implementation at both national (governmental) and local levels often blurs the difference between need and demand, and between science and vested interests.

Case study

Bill's breathlessness and generally poor physical condition is limiting his activity levels (even walking from the work car park to his office is now effortful, particularly if it is windy or humid). His GP is aware that Bill is struggling so has referred him for pulmonary rehabilitation (PR). Bill is quite keen to do this course but the waiting list is months as the number of PR places available does not meet demand. He continues to smoke and does little physical activity so the longer he waits for a place, the more disabled he becomes. He gets very irritated by his cousin, Liam, who also has COPD. Liam lives in Glasgow, he has been on several PR courses, and is forever telling Bill how marvellous they were, and how much more able he feels to manage his COPD symptoms now, and keep off the fags.

Evidence-based guidelines for the management of COPD in adults in primary and secondary care have been set out by NICE in 2010 (**www. nice.org.uk/nicemedia/live/13029/49425/49425.pdf**). If you were Bill's GP, what do you need to know about his COPD in order to provide him with best practice healthcare? Consider the national and international guidelines for COPD (e.g. NICE (**http://guidance.nice.org.uk/ CG101**) and GOLD (**www.goldcopd.com**)) – do these differ?

> ## *Chapter summary*
>
> This chapter provides an introduction to population health. Global patterns of health and healthcare, and the determinants of health, are discussed in the context of public health goals. Epidemiology is defined and briefly explained. Clinical effectiveness and quality improvement tools are discussed, as are planning health services and healthcare decision-making to ensure we have the right type of health services available in the future. The chapter finishes with a brief introduction to health economics and how this can help to inform healthcare planning and decision-making by structured evaluations which make explicit the costs and benefits of health interventions. Examples are given to provide practical illustrations of how epidemiology, health economics and other public health tools underpin clinical guidelines and standards, and hence inform day-to-day medical practice.

GOING FURTHER

Carr, S, Unwin, N and Pless-Mulloli, T (2007) *An Introduction to Public Health and Epidemiology*. Berkshire: Open University Press.
Presents a broad, interactive account of contemporary public health, placing an emphasis on developing public health skills.

Pencheon, D, Guest, C, Melzer, D and Grey, M (eds) (2006) *Oxford Handbook of Public Health Practice*, 2nd edition. Oxford: Oxford University Press.
A practical guide to the practice of public health on a day-to-day basis, suitable for those in training and practice.

Acknowledgement

Our thanks to Mike Crilly, University of Aberdeen, for allowing us to adapt his teaching materials on health needs analysis in this chapter.

chapter 6

Promoting and Improving Health at a Population Level

Cairns Smith and Finlay Dick

Achieving your medical degree

This chapter will help you to meet the following requirements of *Tomorrow's Doctors* (2009).

11 Apply the principles, method and knowledge of population health and the improvement of health and healthcare to your medical practice.

   (e) Explain and apply the basic principles of communicable disease control in hospital and community settings.
   (g) Recognise the role of environmental and occupational hazards in ill health and discuss ways to mitigate their effects.
   (h) Discuss the role of nutrition in health.
   (i) Discuss the principles and application of primary, secondary and tertiary prevention of disease.

Chapter overview

After reading this chapter, you will be able to discuss the following:

* The concepts of health promotion and prevention from a public health perspective, and to show how these are applied in practice, illustrated by
   o communicable disease control measures
   o identifying and mitigating environmental and occupational hazards to health
   o nutrition
* the advantages and disadvantages of different approaches to health promotion.

Introduction

This chapter builds on the concepts and basics of population health outlined in the previous chapter. It is organised in terms of a very broad definition of promoting health, one which encompasses a range of approaches but with a focus on supporting positive health through government, economic and social change rather than individual change (see Chapter 3). The chapter includes discussion of the more clinical aspects of public health around the control of communicable diseases such as, for example, methicillin-resistant *Staphylococcus aureus* (MRSA), avian flu and sexually transmitted infections (STIs) in populations, as well as identifying and addressing occupational and environmental influences on health.

Promoting and improving health

Promoting health is the process of enabling people to increase control over, and to improve, their health. This includes actions directed at both the determinants of health that are outside the immediate control of individuals, including social, economic and environmental conditions, and the determinants within the more immediate control of individuals, including individual health behaviours.

Health is a positive concept emphasising social and personal resources, as well as physical capacities. Therefore, health promotion is not just the responsibility of the health sector, but goes beyond healthy lifestyles to well-being (Ottawa Charter for Health Promotion, 1986). The Ottawa Charter refers to health promotion as quite radical social change, not simply an adjustment in individual lifestyles. The Charter argues that enabling people to gain or increase control over the determinants of their health means challenging the status quo (accepted ways of doing things) at an individual and collective level (community/society). Consequently, health promotion is viewed as something that is not just the remit of the health sector. For example, health promotion activities include government policy to manage a swine flu epidemic, or infection control measures in a hospital, or providing free nicotine replacement therapy, but they also include using money raised through taxation to build a new leisure centre in the community, or using local council power to limit the number of car park spaces at a factory or university to 'force' people to use other, hopefully more healthy means of transport to get to work.

This chapter takes a broad public health view of promoting health, focusing on health promotion at a social, economic and environmental level. You are probably more familiar with the narrower concept of health promotion as educational interventions aimed at particular groups in society. However, health promotion was formerly used as an overarching term which encompassed health education, disease prevention and health protection (Downie *et al.*, 1990).

Disease prevention involves specific interventions aimed at avoiding contact with disease producing risk factors or, where this is not possible, treatment aimed at minimising the harmful consequences of the disease process. It is commonly divided into three levels: primary, secondary and tertiary prevention (see later), and also may involve policy and legislation, such as supporting sports initiatives (e.g. building swimming pools) to enable local populations to do more exercise. A fourth level of health prevention, primordial prevention, has recently been proposed. These are briefly defined below and then discussed in more detail.

Primary prevention: The prevention of the onset of disease in healthy individuals, activities that reduce the risk, severity and duration of disease, illness or injury.

Secondary prevention: Interventions aimed at the early detection and treatment of disease.

Tertiary prevention: Aims to reduce the consequences of disease and disability, and prevent deterioration.

Primordial prevention: A more fundamental level of prevention which addresses the broader social and environmental circumstances that predispose to disease in society.

Health protection involves collective activities directed at factors which are beyond the control of the individual. Health protection activities tend to be regulations or policies, or voluntary codes of practice aimed at the prevention of ill health or the positive enhancement of well-being. A topical health protection activity would be banning smoking in enclosed public places.

Health education is an activity involving communication with individuals or groups aimed at changing knowledge, beliefs, attitudes and behaviour in a direction which is conducive to improvements in health. Thus, health education refers to giving advice and information to an individual or population, e.g. educating teenage girls (a specific population) as to the dangers of smoking to reduce smoking rates in this population or, one-to-one counselling. Health promotion in the form of population health education is discussed briefly in this chapter while individual behaviour change is described in Chapter 3.

Health promotion is used to address major health challenges across the world, including communicable and non-communicable disease and issues related to human development and health. As mentioned earlier in this book, there are certain prerequisites for health that include peace, adequate economic resources (and their distribution), food and shelter, clean water, a stable ecosystem, sustainable resource use and access to basic human rights.

We will now discuss disease prevention, health protection and education in more detail.

Disease prevention

Primary, secondary, tertiary and primordial health prevention

Prevention of disease and reduction in the consequences of disease are major priorities for any health service. Doctors are rightly concerned with diagnosis and treatment of disease, and managing the consequences of disease, but the importance of prevention must not be neglected. Health services, as well as focusing on disease management, must also give priority to interventions aimed at disease prevention. Prevention requires approaches that look beyond people who present with symptoms to those at risk of disease, those with pre-clinical disease and those with impairments and disabilities. The activities to prevent disease, detect early disease and minimise the long-term consequences of disease take place in hospitals, primary care and community settings and are supported by health services, social services, the voluntary sector and families.

Primary prevention

Primary prevention focusses on the prevention of the onset of disease in healthy individuals, activities that reduce the risk, severity and duration of disease, illness or injury. Immunisation is an important form of primary prevention. Immunisation can be given at a population level where all infants are recommended to receive a course of immunisation, which not only protects the individual children but also contributes to a high level of herd immunity, preventing the circulation and transmission of the infectious agent in the community (see Table 6.1). Herd immunity is a concept whereby transmission of an infection ceases when a certain proportion of the population is immune. Immunisation programmes aim to achieve this level, the proportions required vary between infections. The concept is dependent on the uniform uptake of immunisation as clusters of unimmunised, susceptible individuals can present a risk of infection. For example, immunisation against tetanus using tetanus toxoid prevents tetanus in healthy people. This is given as a course of immunisation in infancy and as a booster immunisation in individuals without recent immunisation who are at high risk of tetanus following injury. Immunisation has caused dramatic improvements in health. Because of immunisation, diseases such as diphtheria, tetanus, whooping cough, measles and polio, which used to be major causes of ill health, are now rare in many countries, including the UK (although note that there was a recent [March 2011] outbreak of measles in Leeds, which is an example of what can happen when the immunisation levels drop in a population) (**www. bbc.co.uk/news/uk-england-leeds-12811545**).

Table 6.1 Routine Childhood Immunisation Schedule (UK) January 2011

UK 2011 Immunisation Schedule	
3 days	1. BCG (if there has been tuberculosis in the family in the previous 6 months). 2. Hepatitis B vaccine if mother is HBsAg +ve.
2 months	1. Diphtheria, tetanus, pertussis, polio and *Haemophilus influenzae* type b (DTaP/IPV/Hib). 2. Pneumococcal conjugate vaccine (PCV).
3 months	1. Diphtheria, tetanus, pertussis, polio and *H. influenzae* type b (DTaP/IPV/Hib). 2. Meningitis C (MenC).
4 months	1. Diphtheria, tetanus, pertussis, polio and *H. influenzae* type b (DTaP/IPV/Hib). 2. Pneumococcal conjugate vaccine (PCV). 3. Meningitis C (MenC).
Between 12 and 13 months	1. Measles, mumps and rubella (MMR). 2. Pneumococcal conjugate vaccine (PCV). 3. *H. influenzae* type b, meningitis C (Hib/MenC).
3 years and 4 months to 5 years	1. Diphtheria, tetanus, pertussis and polio (dTaP/IPV or DTaP/IPV). 2. Measles, mumps and rubella (MMR).
Girls aged 12 to 13 years	• Cervical cancer caused by human papillomavirus (HPV) types 16 and 18.
13–18 years	• Tetanus, diphtheria and polio (Td/IPV).

Source: ©EMIS 2011, adapted from **www.patient.co.uk/doctor/Immunisation-Schedule-(UK).htm**, reproduced with permission.

A number of other vaccines are given on a non-routine basis, for example Hepatitis B and BCG at birth for at-risk babies. Immunisation can also be targeted to individuals at increased personal risk such as cholera vaccination for individuals travelling to affected areas, or anthrax vaccine to those working in the leather industry exposed to potentially contaminated skin hides. Passive immunisation may be offered to high-risk individuals such as the immune-suppressed who have been exposed to an infectious agent.

ACTIVITY 6.1

You would no doubt be aware of the recent mumps, measles and rubella (MMR) vaccine controversy. This arose from the claim of a link between the vaccine and autism in a *Lancet* article by Dr Andrew Wakefield. This research has been declared as fraudulent for several reasons (e.g. undeclared interests); Wakefield was found guilty by the General Medical Council (GMC) of serious professional misconduct in May 2010 and was struck off the Medical Register. However, the claims in Wakefield's *Lancet* article were widely reported, and vaccination rates in the UK and Ireland dropped sharply, which in turn led to greatly increased incidence of measles and mumps. What are the potential implications of a substantial drop off in MMR vaccination rates in terms of the individual and herd immunity?

Health education and health promotion interventions aimed at behaviour change such as increased physical activity, smoking cessation or dietary change are also forms of primary prevention when they are applied to healthy people. The use of car seat belts, where healthy individuals have a reduced risk of injury in a road traffic accident or the severity of injury is minimised, can also be considered a primary prevention activity.

ACTIVITY 6.2

A local health authority introduces free membership to local sports facilities to improve the health and fitness of its ageing population.

What would count as evidence that it had worked?

How would you measure improvement?

How would you assess if it provided good value for money?

Secondary prevention

Secondary prevention refers to interventions aimed at the early detection and treatment of disease (to prevent progression). The approach assumes that the early detection of pre-symptomatic disease will lead to more effective treatment, increased survival and reduced consequences of disease. The intervention is usually in the form of a screening programme. For example, breast cancer screening by periodic mammography in women of a specific age range to detect pre-clinical and asymptomatic breast cancer is an example of secondary prevention. Regular self-examination of breasts by women to detect breast lumps is also a form of secondary prevention but it is not considered as effective as regular mammography.

A screening test is not intended to establish a diagnosis with complete certainty. Its purpose is to be able to screen large numbers of people, most of whom will be normal, in order to highlight a smaller proportion of people who may then be referred for more rigorous definitive tests. For example, women with mammographic abnormalities are biopsied to determine those with the disease and those without. Individuals identified as positive on faecal occult blood test as part of colorectal cancer screening are referred for colonoscopy and further investigations before diagnosis and treatment. What a good screening test does (see later for what makes a screening test good) is establish relative risk.

ACTIVITY 6.3

Explaining risks to patients in an effective way is an essential part of ensuring that consent is 'informed'. However, doctors report that they find discussing risk with patients extremely difficult. This might be related to the fact that doctors use statistical models of risk (e.g. a 70-year-old male smoker with high blood pressure has an xx per cent risk of a cardiovascular event in the next five years) while patients tend to see themselves as high or low risk generally, and also use concepts such as luck and destiny, and the views of friends, neighbours and the media, in their assessment of personal risk (Paling, 2003).

Screening can be organised at a population level in national programmes or can be conducted opportunistically when individuals present for other reasons. Thus, some screening programmes are targeted at individuals considered to be at high risk of a disease such as glaucoma screening for people who have first-degree relatives with glaucoma. In certain occupational setting, screening may be adopted where a number of conditions are screened for at the sample time such as blood pressure, blood cholesterols and urine analysis for sugar (a more opportunistic approach to screening). In national screening programmes apparently healthy individuals are identified, often from list of patients registered with the NHS or with general practitioners, and are invited to attend for a screening examination on a call and recall basis (see below) to achieve a high level of population coverage.

There are a number of different national screening programmes such as cervical cancer, breast cancer and colorectal cancer programmes. National screening

---

Call and recall

The NHS Call and Recall System holds a list of all patients registered with a GP in the area it covers. This system sends the list of people due for screening (e.g. women due for cervical screening) to each GP to check the records (for correct name and address and in case it is not appropriate for them to be invited). The Call and Recall System sends the list of patients checked by the GP the invitation letters and reminder letters, and the result letter from the screening.

---

programmes are usually expensive and labour-intensive and are carefully audited at practice, regional and national levels.

There is often public, political and media pressure to start new screening programmes. So why not just have screening tests for all common diseases? There is more to screening than just how many people have a disease: it is important to critically appraise whether certain criteria are met. The criteria used to decide whether or not a screening programme will be worthwhile were originally proposed by Wilson and Jungner (1968).

Characteristics of the disease:	• The disease must be an important public health problem. • The natural history of the disease should be adequately understood. • The disease must have a clinically detectable pre-symptomatic phase.	
Characteristics of the test:	The test must be:	- valid, i.e. sensitive and specific. - safe. - acceptable to both the public and professionals.
Characteristics of the treatment:	The treatment must be:	- of proven effectiveness. - relatively safe. - acceptable to both the public and professionals.
Considerations of organisation and cost:	• Facilities for diagnosis and treatment should be available. • There should be an agreed policy on who to treat as patients, and how to manage borderline cases. • Screening needs to be a continuing process. • The economic cost of the programme should not be unreasonably high.	

Figure 6.1 Adapted from Wilson and Jungner's (1968) criteria for assessing a screening test.

Wilson and Jungner refer to sensitivity and specificity. The screening test must be sensitive (give positive results in those with disease) and specific (give negative results in those without disease). It is important that the screening test avoids false-positives (creating anxiety in the healthy individuals) and false-negatives (wrongly reassuring individuals who have the disease). Wilson and Jungner's criteria have been recently updated by the World Health Organization (**www.who.int/bulletin/volumes/86/4/07-050112/en**; Andermann *et al.*, 2008).

WHO synthesis of emerging screening criteria proposed over the past 40 years:

- The screening programme should respond to a recognised need.
- The objectives of screening should be defined at the outset.
- There should be a defined target population.
- There should be scientific evidence of screening programme effectiveness.
- The programme should integrate education, testing, clinical services and programme management.
- There should be quality assurance, with mechanisms to minimise potential risks of screening.
- The programme should ensure informed choice, confidentiality and respect for autonomy.
- The programme should promote equity and access to screening for the entire target population.
- Programme evaluation should be planned from the outset.
- The overall benefits of screening should outweigh the harm.

Screening programmes may meet the criteria for national implementation, for selective implementation for specific high-risk groups, for use in an opportunistic approach or not meet the criteria for implementation at any level.

ACTIVITY 6.4

Doctors working in general practice surgeries tend to meet either those who are already ill and for whom prevention is perhaps too late or the middle class 'worried well' who are less likely to experience premature mortality. Of course, ceasing smoking at any age will benefit the health of the individual concerned but how do you direct preventive services to those most likely to experience preventable illnesses and diseases? Specifically, how would you go about identifying current smokers from practice records, how would you approach the discussion about smoking cessation with them? You may find Chapters 3 and 7 useful in terms of informing how you would do this.

Tertiary prevention

Tertiary prevention aims to reduce the consequences of disease and disability, and prevent deterioration (in other words, minimise the damage of a disease). Much of the work of health services is tertiary prevention aimed at limiting disability and enhancing quality of life in individuals with disease. Joint replacement in individuals whose joints have been damaged by severe arthritis improves mobility, reduces pain and enhances quality of life: this is an example of tertiary prevention. Another example of tertiary prevention is rehabilitation for people with COPD or after stroke.

Tertiary prevention is the most medical/clinical level of prevention as it includes giving treatment to prevent a disease from spreading. Medication could be steroids for asthma (to prevent asthma attacks) or prescribing beta-blockers to patients with high blood pressure (to prevent strokes).

Primordial prevention

Primordial prevention is a more fundamental level of prevention which addresses the broader social and environmental circumstances that pre-dispose to disease in society. The clear distinction between primordial and primary prevention relates to primordial prevention activities lying outside the doctor–patient relationship and the medical model. It calls for changing the socio-economic status of society as better socio-economic status correlates inversely with lifestyle factors such as smoking, abnormal food patterns and exercise. Thus, examples of primordial prevention would be a government subsidising certain commodities, like basic food stuffs, or taxing other goods, such as tobacco and alcohol. It is a relatively new concept which is receiving attention in the prevention of chronic diseases as many adult chronic diseases (e.g. obesity, hypertension) are now known to have their origin in childhood.

The hypothesis of the 'thrifty phenotype' (Hales and Barker, 1992), or the foetal programming hypothesis, is relevant here. This hypothesis proposes that reduced foetal growth, due to poor maternal nutrition, is strongly associated with a number of chronic conditions later in life, including coronary heart disease, stroke, diabetes and hypertension. Why is this? It seems that if the mother has an inadequate diet then it signals the baby that the living condition in the long term will be impoverished. Consequently the baby adapts by reducing its body size and metabolism to prepare for harsh conditions of food shortages after birth. When the living environment switches from the condition of malnutrition to a society of abundant supply of nutrients, this exposes the baby to an environment that goes against what its body is designed for and this places the baby at a higher risk of metabolic adult diseases later in adulthood. In short, maternal malnutrition may be a cause of increased disease susceptibility in her baby in adulthood. Political, environmental and socio-economic factors need to be addressed to ensure adequate nutrition for all and hence primordial prevention (e.g. improving the supply of nutritious food) is one approach to improving health in the population.

Health protection

As mentioned earlier in this chapter, health protection involves collective activities directed at factors which are beyond the control of the individual. Legislation that ends smoking in workplaces and public places both eliminate exposure to second-hand smoke, which increases the risk of myocardial infarction, and reduces the prevalence of smoking and cigarette consumption. A national strategy to respond to an infectious disease outbreak could also be considered health protection. Health protection activities tend to be regulations or policies, or voluntary codes of practice aimed at the prevention of ill health or the positive enhancement of well-being.

Control of infectious diseases

An example of health protection in which public health doctors have a specific role is the control of infectious diseases. Disease control is defined as interventions to reduce the incidence or the prevalence of a disease in a population. Disease elimination is a term used to define programmes aiming to reduce the incidence of a disease to a pre-defined very low level and eradication to the level where no new diseases occur.

NICE provides guidance on healthcare-associated infection in primary and community care (**http://guidance.nice.org.uk/CG2**). Those of you studying in Scotland will be familiar with 'Cleanliness Champions', an educational programme aimed at infection control, part of the work of the Scottish Government's approach to reducing healthcare-associated infection within NHS Scotland.

The principles of disease control in hospitals and community settings are similar; however the environments and those involved will be different. The key principles are surveillance, preventive measures and outbreak management.

Surveillance

Communicable diseases are no longer a major cause of death in Western countries but they do contribute to considerable morbidity and have an economic impact through days lost to work. In low-income countries, communicable diseases remain a major cause of both morbidity and mortality. The patterns of communicable diseases are continually changing with new communicable diseases emerging such as Lyme disease and HIV infection and many older diseases such as tuberculosis (TB) and syphilis re-emerging in certain circumstances (e.g. multi-drug resistance, the interaction between different infections such as TB and HIV).

The patterns of communicable diseases are the result of the interactions between the infectious agent, the host and the environment. The source of infection may be human, there may be animal reservoirs such as brucellosis in cattle or leptospirosis in rats, or reservoirs of infection may exist in the environment in water or soil.

There are a number of modes of transmission between the source and the host through direct or indirect transmission (by vectors or vehicles). Vehicles such as water (for example cryptosporidiosis) or food (salmonellosis) carry the infective agent while vectors such as mosquitoes for malaria are part of the life cycle. The transmission of infection may be by inhalation, ingestion, direct skin or mucosal contact, sexual contact, injection or cross-placental routes. The susceptibility of the host is influenced by age, natural immunity, artificial immunity (active or passive), nutritional status and immune suppression.

The classical method of surveillance of communicable diseases is through a process of notification. Specific infections are deemed to be notifiable and doctors suspecting such infections are legally required to notify public health authorities. Different countries have different lists and the system may not be very responsive and can be potentially stigmatising for individuals. Commonly the notification systems use telephone and electronic systems where urgent notification is required.

More rapid and comprehensive methods of surveillance use microbiology laboratory reports of infections to trigger action required to protect the public. Sentinel systems of surveillance (ongoing systematic collection, analysis and interpretation of data and the distribution of this data to those who need to know) are commonly used to monitor conditions presenting at a primary healthcare level such as influenza.

Surveillance systems operate locally through the NHS health protection teams and the information is aggregated and reported at national levels on a weekly basis. There are regional and international networks for surveillance and the WHO produces a Weekly Epidemiological Record at a global level. Surveillance is important in recognising the background frequency of communicable diseases so that changes in incidence over time and outbreaks can be identified. The surveillance information is also used to monitor the impact of interventions such as immunisations. There is also routine surveillance of the uptake of intervention measures such as immunisations where uptake rates are assessed for different target groups to ensure that the target uptake rates are achieved geographically and in specific socio-economic and high-risk groups.

ACTIVITY 6.5

What possible problems do you foresee in a public health notification system which has the effect that it stigmatises individuals with a particular disease or infection? (A stigma has been defined as a discrediting attribute which taints and can denigrate a person. For example, society might look down on people with a mental illness, drug misuse problems or a sexually transmitted infection (STI) and treat them differently than people without such disease.)

Preventive measures

Preventive measures for communicable disease are aimed at reducing exposures of the populations to the agents of infection and at increasing the host immunity to specific infections.

There is a wide range of prevention measures to protect populations from exposure to infectious agents and to reduce the risk of communicable diseases. These include measures to prevent exposure to water and food borne diseases, as well as wider environmental interventions to minimise exposures. Local government and water authorities are required to ensure safe water distribution through a range of water treatment systems and routine water quality assessments at different points through the water distribution systems. Environmental agencies have responsibility for the protection of water systems from various forms of environmental contamination. Animal husbandry, veterinary practice and food safety measures are required to minimise the risk of exposure to food-borne diseases. Environmental health authorities of local government have responsibilities for education and inspection of food premises to ensure food safety.

Infections (healthcare-associated infections) in a hospital setting are very important as up to 10 per cent of patients may acquire infection in a hospital. The commonest are urinary infection, respiratory infection, wound infection and septicaemia. A number of organisms have acquired resistance to antibiotics such as methicillin-resistant *Staphylococcus aureus* (MRSA). Preventive measures specific to hospital settings must take account of the nature of procedures being undertaken, the potential of specific antibiotic resistance organisms, and the presence of highly susceptible individuals with significant co-morbidities and altered immune status. There are standard protocols for all procedures to minimise the risk of infection and cross-infection; these need to be system-wide approaches as no single measure alone is adequate. Measures include recommendations about personal protective equipment (specialised clothing or equipment worn by an employee for protection against infection), clothing, uniforms, hand washing, disposable equipment, patient isolation, use of antibiotics, cleaning, hospital design and the monitoring of adherence to these recommendations that apply to all hospital users, including medical students. There is mandatory monitoring of MRSA and *Clostridium difficile* infections as well as surveillance of antibiotic use and surgical site infection.

Outbreak investigation and control

Outbreaks occur when there is a change in the balance between the host, the agent, and the environment. Prevention is of prime importance and an outbreak often represents a failure of preventive measures. Routine surveillance of the background levels of infection is essential to establish the endemicity and to help identify the presence of an outbreak. An outbreak is defined as a local increase in the numbers of the specific condition compared to the background endemic level.

The first stage is to confirm the presence of an outbreak, the threshold for action will depend on the severity of the specific condition or the immediate risk to a large number of people. For example, the threshold for investigation for food-borne disease is usually two or more linked cases with the same illness. There may be special settings which need to be considered including hospitals, schools, care homes, prisons or hotels. The next stage is to define the diagnosis which may be a specific infection but in some circumstances a case definition based on a set of signs and symptoms may be used where no organism has yet been identified. Attempts are then made to define the population exposed, to identify any additional cases and to collect information on cases in terms of time of onset, place and the persons affected. An epidemic curve is then plotted using the time of onset of each case (see Figure 6.2). The plot can indicate whether there is a point source (a source common to all victims [e.g. a polluted water outlet] where the exposure occurs in less than one incubation period) or a propagated curve (indicating person to person transmission; note that a continuing point source can have a similar plot to a propagated curve). Identification of the organism and its known incubation period can allow estimation of when the exposure took place. Further analysis can be conducted using case–control or cohort methods (see Chapter 7) to test a hypothesis.

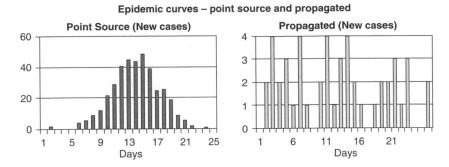

Figure 6.2 An epidemic curve – point source and propagated.

A vital part in the management of any outbreak is to instigate preventive measures to minimise the risk of further exposure. This may take the form of closing food premises, withdrawing items from sale or replacing water supplies. Interventions such as immunisation (for example, rabies) and chemoprophylaxis (meningococcal disease) can be used when at-risk exposed individuals have been identified. The interventions, where appropriate, must be instituted as soon as possible. Examples of outbreaks in hospital settings would include MRSA and *C. difficile*. Infections which are more likely to have a community origin include severe acute respiratory syndrome (SARS) and avian flu. For any infection, there are protocols for minimising the risk of further exposure, including how to effectively manage infected patients in hospital.

Outbreak investigation and management is usually conducted by an outbreak, or infection, control team led by a consultant in public health. The membership of the outbreak control team will vary according to the nature of the outbreak but often includes public health nurses, clinical microbiologists and environmental health officers.

An infection control team would typically do the following:

- Provide an advice service for staff to help them prevent and manage infection. Advise on the management of individual patients, or on clusters or outbreaks of infection. Provide advice about decontamination of equipment and the environment, or about best practice in the prevention of infection associated with any area of healthcare.

- Conduct a programme of audit (environment and practice) and surveillance.

- Produce guidelines for all staff on the prevention and management of infection.

- Provide input to the education programmes provided by the trust for all staff.

- Be involved in research to improve infection control practice.

- Liaise with staff involved in purchasing and planning to ensure infection control issues are given a high priority in their activities.

- Liaise with other departments to provide infection control input, e.g. occupational health, catering.

- Communicate with the media.

Health education

Health education is the development of individual, group, institutional, community and systemic strategies to improve health knowledge, attitudes, skills and behaviour. The purpose of health education is to positively influence the health behaviour of individuals and communities as well as the living and working conditions that influence their health.

ACTIVITY 6.6

Go to the UK Department of Health's website, and search for 'health education and promotion'. You will find an enormous number of resources covering a range of topics from hand hygiene to alcohol awareness, from using mobile phones to a guide to healthy fasting, from eating five portions of fruit and vegetables a day, and so on. Choose one of these resources to read in more depth, and consider this reading in relation to your own behaviour.

Health education includes written materials (e.g. the leaflets you pick up at your GP surgery or pharmacy), TV advertisements (e.g. be alert to carbon monoxide dangers), lectures and talks (e.g. sexual awareness and use of contraception to senior school pupils).

ACTIVITY 6.7

Many doctors are extremely cynical about health education/promotion and question if the resources allocated to it are money well spent. Stop and think for a moment about your own reactions to health promotion advertisements, for example contraception and AIDS, eat five portions of fruit and vegetables a day. Do you think health promotions adverts have any influence on your own behaviour?

Unfortunately, it is difficult to adequately evaluate the majority of health education/promotion activities because of the complexities surrounding attempts to achieve long-term behaviour change and the need to devote further resources to developing appropriate methods for its evaluation. Naidoo and Wills (2005) argue that three aspects of health promotion campaigns should be evaluated:

1. Efficiency – to assess what has been achieved and whether an intervention had the intended effect.

2. Effectiveness – to measure its impact and whether it was worthwhile.

3. Economy – to judge its cost-effectiveness and whether time, money and labour were well spent.

These can be relatively easily assessed with screening where specificity and sensitivity can be measured but less so with a health intervention aimed at increasing fruit and vegetable consumption or fitness. With many different interested parties and possible outcomes, a more pluralistic approach to evaluation is needed involving a number of criteria and evaluation methods.

Environmental and occupational hazards in ill health

Occupational and environmental medicine operates within the concept of the environment as a determinant of health and disease. This includes atmospheric and ecological influences as well as factors such as society, housing and work. As its basis, it takes a positive view of health and examines how people relate to their environment and adapt either the environment or themselves when necessary. When the process of adaptation is inappropriate or impossible, remedial action must be taken.

Environmental influences on health were introduced in Chapter 1, along with the basic concepts of hazard and risk, and the interaction between individual and environmental factors.

Environmental influences on health are discussed in more detail in this chapter as occupational and environmental medicine works at several different levels to protect health: from population, to group, to the individual. There are many examples of health education, protection and prevention in occupational and environmental medicine.

Exposure

Before discussing this topic in more depth, you need to know a little about the concept of exposure. Exposure to a pollutant (such as paint fumes at work, poor air quality in the wider environment) should be measured both in terms of level and duration. Some pollutants act immediately in producing adverse health outcomes, such as in the London smog example given in Chapter 1. Others produce effects only after prolonged exposure (e.g. radiation, lead) such as the Chernobyl nuclear accident. When trying to establish the relationship between exposure and an environmental pollutant, it is important to quantify as accurately as possible the level and duration of exposure needed to produce a health effect. It is often easier to identify occupational exposures which lead to ill health as illness occurs within defined groups of employees who share similar exposures, for example to lead, asbestos, paint fumes and airborne allergens. Environmental exposures are generally one or two orders of magnitude lower than those found in the workplace, but occur for longer and those exposed include vulnerable groups such as the elderly, the young and the infirm. Not infrequently hazards are first recognised among workers and only later identified as also being environmental hazards.

Exposure pathways

The environment is often considered as the outdoor space we occupy but, in terms of health, environmental exposures may occur through the air we breathe, the food we eat, the water we drink (see 'What's the evidence?' below) and the soil on which we walk. There is much interest in outdoor air quality in the Western world but the global health burden of high indoor smoke from burning biomass fuels such as wood and charcoal is much greater. Globally, poor indoor air quality affects over 3 billion people and causes almost 2 million deaths per year.

What's the evidence?

In the 1960s and 1970s, efforts to provide microbiologically safe drinking water led to the drilling of many wells in the Indian sub-continent. Sadly, no one thought to test these wells for contamination with metals. Had they done so high levels of arsenic would have been found as the underlying rocks are arsenic-rich. This led to the largest mass poisoning in human history with over 20 million people in Bangladesh and West Bengal affected. Health effects included hyperpigmentation, skin hyperkeratosis and skin, bladder and pancreatic cancer. Control measures include educating the populace about arsenic, closing the most contaminated wells, sand filtration of contaminated water and harvesting uncontaminated rainwater.

This example also demonstrates the different levels of response to the harm caused by the contaminated water – population group (education) and governmental/community (addressing the problem at its source).

In the workplace, the primary route of exposure is via inhalation with skin exposure being a secondary route; skin irritants/allergens and chemicals such as some pesticides are readily absorbed by the skin. Ingestion is an unusual exposure route in the work setting (but not in the home where most accidental poisonings are due to ingestion) although practices such as nail biting can lead to significant ingestion of workplace contaminants. Injection is a minor pathway for workplace exposure except in certain occupations such as healthcare workers (e.g. needlestick injuries; see also Chapter 1).

Poor training, maintenance and regulation, both in factories and the wider environment, can also contribute to harm in the form of accidents. Every year tens of thousands of people around the world are injured or lose their lives in accidents. Workplace accidents are commonest in construction, mining and agriculture and are more likely where safety controls are lax or absent. Most workplace accidents only affect workers but the public are also at risk. Examples of such accidents include a chemical leak in a pesticide factory in Bhopal, India, which is thought to have killed 3800 people and injured 15,000 and the Chernobyl nuclear disaster in the Ukraine, which killed 50 people in its immediate aftermath and forced the evacuation of over

350,000 people. Non-occupational accidents are commoner in the developing world where poor standards of construction and maintenance and poor transport safety add to the burden of accidents.

Exposure measurement and assessment

It is not enough to recognise that a hazard to human health exists: to effectively control the hazard requires an understanding of the agent and how exposure to it is occurring. This requires assessment and, where possible, measurement of exposures. A particular challenge in dealing with environmental exposures can be obtaining a sufficiently large sample of the agent for meaningful analysis.

Exposure control

Governments can play an important part in controlling both environmental and workplace hazards, for example, by passing laws regarding health and safety at work. However, without enforcement, such legislation may be ineffective.

For employers, the first step to controlling workplace hazards is hazard recognition. Having identified that a hazard exists, and that it poses a risk to health, measures to reduce the risk to an acceptable level are necessary. In an occupational setting, the approach to controlling such risks may involve substitution of a less hazardous agent or process; engineering controls; administrative controls; and, sometimes, personal protective equipment. Examples of substitution include using toluene as a solvent instead of benzene (which causes leukaemia) and using welding instead of riveting as riveting exposes the worker to the risk of both hand-arm vibration syndrome and noise-induced hearing loss. Engineering controls cover such measures as enclosing dusty machines; fitting silencers on noisy compressors; and improving workplace ventilation. Roof-mounted fans are one example of general exhaust ventilation. While these are appropriate for nuisance dusts, they are ineffective for controlling toxic chemicals or dusts: these must be captured at source using local exhaust ventilation (LEV). The laboratory fume cupboard is one example of LEV. Administrative controls include task rotation to reduce musculoskeletal problems; worker training; and restricting access to hazardous areas. Finally, personal protective equipment such as gloves, face masks or ear defenders may be used where other measures are insufficient to control hazards. Such equipment is a last line of defence as it can only work when worn.

Where exposures occur, effective control may require action by government as well as by organisations and individuals. Thus, in the UK, workplaces must adhere to certain government rules and regulations designed to limit hazards and accidents.

ACTIVITY 6.8

Search for the Health and Safety Executive (HSE) online (**www.hse.gov.uk**). This is a governmental agency whose mission is to prevent death, injury and ill-health in Britain's workplaces. The website is very comprehensive, providing guidance for employers (e.g. government regulations for storing dangerous substances) and individuals (e.g. how to prevent and treat health issues such as back pain and stress). Search for the HSE advice on how to prevent back injury, a very common occupational health issue in the NHS.

However, recognising that a hazard exists does not necessarily translate into regulatory action. For example, firearms deaths are much commoner in the USA than in most European countries, in part reflecting Americans' easier access to guns, but gun control has proven a highly contentious issue in America where the right to bear arms is enshrined in the second amendment. Measures which can be taken to control environmental hazards include better regulation of industry and in particular control of industrial discharges into the air and water and improved waste management. Chemical works, mines and other industrial sites can cause ill health in neighbouring communities by contaminating their air, water and soil. Human exposure may then occur by multiple pathways due to breathing contaminated air, drinking contaminated water (see 'What's the evidence?') and eating food which itself has been contaminated.

Recognition of environmental or occupational illness

If you are to make a diagnosis of an occupational or environmental illness, then you must first consider this possibility. Broadly speaking, there are three ways in which such issues come to light:

- a cluster of disease in a workforce or community;
- recognition of high exposures leading to surveys of exposed populations;
- by analogy with other recognised exposure/response relationships.

Where occupational or environmental illness is suspected, a detailed history should be taken. Investigation of the workplace or wider environment requires specific skills and the advice of experts, such as exposure scientists, may be required to quantify exposures. Having identified an occupational or environmental disease, action is needed not just to treat the individual cases but to protect public health by introducing control measures such as those listed above to prevent further illness.

Case study

There are no data to show conclusively that screening spirometry is effective in directing management decisions or in improving COPD outcomes in patients who are identified before the development of significant symptoms. However, a GP with a special interest in COPD employed a medical student over the summer to carry out a case-finding exercise. This involved sending all smokers older than 40 a questionnaire asking about symptoms such as cough and wheeze. On the basis of his responses to this questionnaire, Bill was invited in to the practice for a spirometry test to check poor bronchodilator reversibility, and a full social and occupational history was taken by his GP. This indicated that, as well as being a life-long smoker, he had worked in an enclosed environment with low ceilings and poor ventilation for many years when he was a 'hands-on' baker, before the introduction of UK health and safety regulations for ventilation.

Bill was diagnosed with COPD. Consequently, in line with guideline recommendations, he is receiving tertiary prevention in the form of medication (anticholinergic bronchodilators) and annual flu vaccinations to prevent further exacerbations. He has also been advised to stop smoking and was offered counselling and nicotine replacement therapy, but he has not quit yet.

Chapter summary

This chapter has introduced various population health approaches to improving health and healthcare, specifically health promotion and education, and prevention. Many clinical examples were provided to illustrate these approaches in practice. This chapter also covered exposure, exposure pathways, measure, protection and control in relation to infectious disease and environmental and occupational hazards in ill health.

GOING FURTHER

Naidoo, J and Wills, J (2010) *Developing Practice for Public Health and Health Promotion: Developing Practice*, 3rd edition. London: Bailliere-Tindale.
An introductory book, which focusses on developing knowledge, skills and confidence in these topics.

Levy, BS, Wegman, DH, Baron, SL and Sokas, RK (2011) *Occupational and Environmental Health: Recognizing and Preventing Disease and Injury*, 6th edition. Oxford: Oxford University Press.
Provides comprehensive coverage and a clear understanding of occupational and environmental health and its relationships to public health, environmental science, and governmental policy.

part 2

Applying Knowledge to Clinical Practice

chapter 7

Scientific Method and Critical Appraisal
Philip Cotton and Lindsey Pope

Achieving your medical degree

This chapter will help you to meet the following requirements of *Tomorrow's Doctors* (2009).

11 Apply to medical practice the principles, method and knowledge of population health and the improvement of health and healthcare.

(f) Evaluate and apply epidemiological data in managing healthcare for the individual and the community.

12 Apply scientific method and approaches to medical research.

(a) Critically appraise the results of relevant diagnostic, prognostic and treatment trials and other qualitative and quantitative studies as reported in the medical and scientific literature.
(b) Formulate simple relevant research questions in biomedical science, psychosocial science or population science, and design appropriate studies or experiments to address the questions.
(c) Apply findings from the literature to answer questions raised by specific clinical problems.
(d) Understand the ethical and governance issues involved in medical research.

This chapter introduces some of the key concepts of research study design and critical appraisal. It will help you develop an understanding of how to answer questions raised by clinical problems, read a paper and interpret research findings, as well as how to design a research study, and how research contributes to clinical best practice guidelines. It introduces some key skills and techniques to ensure your own best practice, including research design, audit and reflection.

Chapter overview

After reading this chapter, you will be able to discuss the following:

- How to seek answers to questions in clinical practice.
- How we judge clinical research.
- How we strive for best practice.
- Principal research methods.
- The role of audit in clinical practice.
- The role of reflection in practice.

Questions in practice

Learning in medicine takes place in many different settings. Your own learning will be driven by many experiences and questions. These questions may come from:

- case studies in the curriculum, in lectures or tutorials or self-study or group work;
- visits to clinical environments, in hospital and the community;
- active involvement in clinical teams;
- from your own life, and news reports.

For example, you may wonder whether Emergency Department (ED) triage works, whether telephone consulting is acceptable to patients, and why people in lower social classes smoke more. These are fairly rudimentary questions and your own questions may be much more complex. You might develop these questions into something more explicit and appropriate to your information needs and knowledge gaps, and begin to ask questions about, for example, what happens if someone's condition deteriorates once they have been triaged – is the triage category re-assessed after waiting a period of time in the ED? Formulating and articulating questions like this requires certain knowledge and skills if you are to be successful in finding an answer.

The next sections will take you through some of the typical, and accepted, ways of doing so. These include:

- using existing sources of evidence (databases, primary sources such as journal articles, secondary sources such as guidelines);
- carrying out your own research;
- comparing your own and your colleagues' practice to existing standards (audit).

Existing sources of evidence

To answer questions generated in practice, doctors speak to colleagues, consult textbooks, attend conferences and clinical meetings, turn to journals and other hard-copy sources of evidence, and search regarded websites.

Internet

Increasing numbers of people, including doctors and medical students, access health information on the internet through popular search engines. However, this information is of variable quality and usefulness. Healthcare professionals must familiarise themselves with searchable information sources and databases that they can trust for evidence-based decision-making, and for directing patients to once they leave the clinic.

These might include NHS sites, 'GP notebook', disease-specific professional society sites (e.g. the British Thoracic Society, **www.brit-thoracic.org.uk**) and practitioner sites such as 'tripdatabase' or those of the Royal Colleges (e.g. **www.rcgp.org.uk www.rcpath.org**), or research and national guideline sites (of which more later).

ACTIVITY 7.1

Think about the information needs that arise in your medical studies. Where do you go for information? Do you use popular search engines and open the first few sites that are generated? How do you know whether the sites generated are reliable and accurate? What criteria do you use to decide whether or not a site is trustworthy – or do you accept everything you find on the net as accurate?

Think of the same issues from the perspective of a patient. What issues might arise if the patient's source of information is not trustworthy and evidence-based? For example, if a patient comes to see you with an article cut out of a newspaper, convinced they have a certain disease/illness, but you are equally convinced this is not the case, how would you manage the consultation? Patients also come to clinics with evidence of a 'cure' for their illness with an expectation that you will be able to help them to access this cure.

Hard-copy sources of evidence

These include textbooks and journal articles. Textbooks are extremely useful for medical students as they provide an overview and basic information on the topic under study. With rapid advances in science and knowledge, clinical textbooks need to be updated regularly to reflect new evidence and changing practice.

Journal articles are current – they tell you what is happening right now. However, you need to be able to judge the relevance of an information source to your information need. This is similar to the argument about web sites and includes the question – how can you trust your source of information? Key points when trying to identify a relevant and reliable journal article relate to the journal itself and then the specific article.

In terms of the journal itself, if you are looking for a scholarly article, you search in journals which:

- are academic or professional (who publishes the journal? The BMJ group or a national medical society versus Joe Blogg's home publishing?).

- are peer-reviewed (a process of evaluation where papers are reviewed prepublication by qualified individuals in the field to maintain standards and provide credibility).

- probably have an impact factor (a measure of how many times articles from a journal have been quoted by other researchers in a given period of time – the higher the impact factor the better).

We say probably in relation to the last point as, for example, a new journal, which may publish excellent articles, will not have an impact factor as 'earning' one takes a few years.

Journal home pages will provide all this information.

Let's assume you have identified a number of articles from reputable journals which address your question. How do you then read these articles critically, to know whether or not they might affect the way you think about clinical practice? To do so, you need some basic knowledge about research study design and methods. This basic knowledge will be introduced first, then how this knowledge helps you to read papers will be explained.

Scientific method and approaches

Before setting out on any research study, it is critical to formulate a clear research question: what it is you wish to know before setting out on a search for answers? Defining your specific question helps you make sure it has not already been answered (which you would identify by doing a thorough literature review). If it has not, then a clear question helps you identify the most appropriate study methods, or design, to answer your question.

A research question can be cast as a hypothesis or statement that you set out to prove or disprove. For example, the question 'does drug X give benefits to patients with exacerbations of COPD?' could be cast as a hypothesis along the lines of 'adding in drug X reduces the rate of hospitalisation for exacerbations of COPD'. The question – and the hypothesis – provide the basis for developing a research study.

The answer to the original question about drug X and exacerbations of COPD might exist in the literature. In order to carry out an efficient search of relevant databases, the PICO framework can be useful in formulating certain types of searchable questions. The mnemonic PICO represents People or Patients, Intervention, Comparison, and Outcome of interest and becomes: in people with moderate COPD (P) does adding drug X (I) as opposed to adding nothing (C) reduce the rate of readmission (O).

Your interest might have arisen because you followed a particular patient during his hospitalisation and you are concerned that he hates taking medication, and thus is unlikely to be compliant with a medication regimen. If, after your literature search, you discover that the drug X makes 'little difference' to the readmission rate for people with the same severity of COPD as your patient, you might question whether adding this drug to his daily routine will be a useful intervention for this particular patient anyway.

Research methods

Research methods are used to gather the data which is used as the basis for inference and interpretation, explanation and prediction. The method(s) chosen are guided by the aims of the study (see below for an example of different study aims and appropriate research methods to fulfil these aims).

Research methods are broadly categorised in terms of whether they generate quantitative or qualitative data. Quantitative methods tend to generate numerical data while qualitative methods tend to generate language data (written or oral), although this is not always strictly the case. The choice of research method depends largely on your research question. Clinical research has traditionally used quantitative approaches to answer important questions such as: *is this treatment or intervention effective?* Randomised controlled trials (RCTs, see later) are most appropriate in these circumstances. In recent years, however, qualitative approaches, which seek answers to the 'what', 'how' or 'why' of a phenomenon rather than questions about 'how many?' or 'how much?', are being increasingly used in the health services research, often in combination with quantitative approaches (mixed methods research). For example, if you wish to know whether a new drug can offer an additional benefit to patients in terms of symptom control then an RCT is best. However, if you wish to find out what factors influence recovery after a stroke, you may wish to interview people who have had a stroke to seek their views on the impact of supportive and caring family members. In qualitative research, the research question is exploratory rather than explanatory.

In this next section, some widely used types of research method are described in relation to the type of research questions they can be used to address. (There is not space to provide a comprehensive overview of research methods here so further reading is suggested at the end of the chapter.)

The randomised controlled trial

An experiment is set up to answer a specific question. The question is posed as a hypothesis – that is, it is hypothesised that drug X reduces the incidence of a stroke in woman older than 75 years with no other illnesses. If the experiment gives results that confirm the hypothesis, then this may be presented as evidence for the use of drug X. It is essential that there is nothing in the way in which the experiment is performed that can cause the result seen. Furthermore, there is biological variation between people and so it is important that this is accounted for too.

The challenge for the researchers includes: how to reduce the effect of the result occurring due to chance; how to account for biological variation; and how to ensure that the only difference between two groups of people is the intervention in the research study, e.g. drug X.

The pre-requirements for a randomised trial are that there must be genuine uncertainty, and that there must be informed consent (see later for further discussion).

The features of a randomised controlled trial include the following:

- An appropriate sample of a representative study population.

- Participants are allocated randomly to each 'treatment' group, typically 'new treatment' and 'control' which may be 'placebo' and/or 'current treatment'.

- The double-blind design (triple-blind if possible).

- There is an objective measure of outcome.

- The follow-up of participants is complete.
- The only difference between the groups of participants is the exposure to the intervention.

See Figure 7.1 for the basic structure of a randomised trial.

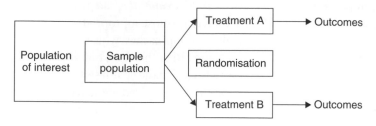

Figure 7.1 The basic structure of a randomised controlled trial.

ACTIVITY 7.2

Research terms like 'randomised controlled trial' and 'double-blind' may be new to you. Using your preferred search engine, find a reputable website such as a medical dictionary, to identify the meanings of the following common research concepts in quantitative research:

- Randomised controlled trial
  - Pragmatic randomised controlled trial
- 'Gold standard'
- Null hypothesis
- Randomisation
  - Random sampling
  - Random allocation
- Single-blind, double-blind, triple-blind
- Placebo, placebo-controlled study
- Intention to treat (ITT) or pragmatic analysis
- Explanatory analysis

Definitions of terms used in epidemiology, in clinical trials, in diagnosis, in statistics, and in health economics can be found on the 'Bandolier' website: **www. medicine.ox.ac.uk/bandolier/glossary.html**

Double-blind randomised controlled trials are considered to be the gold standard research method for testing the benefits of one treatment against another. Participants (patients) are randomly allocated to control or for intervention of study groups, which are closely matched for factors that might affect outcome (e.g. gender, age, stage of disease). However, there are also disadvantages to RCTs:

- RCTs are costly and difficult to set up and run, and hence time-consuming.

- Recruits may not be typical patients (selection bias).

- RCTs cannot address all research questions (e.g. the role of diet in heart disease).

- RCTs are necessarily limited to people who consent to take part and who do not have the exclusion criteria, and, thus, the results of an RCT may not be applicable to all patients.

- Small RCTs may lead to false-negative conclusions (e.g. individual trials may be too small to detect statistically significant results).

The cohort study

In clinical research, a cohort study is a longitudinal, observational study. It is an analysis of risk factors and follows a group of people who do not have the disease under question, and uses correlations to determine the absolute risk of subject contraction of this disease. A cohort study is typically prospective and is used to explore prognosis. A case–control study is usually retrospective (existing data is gathered from medical or other records and analysed and groups are defined after analysis). Prospective cohort studies between exposure and disease strongly aid in studying causal associations.

Figure 7.2 shows a 2 × 2 model. The columns separate people into two groups – those with the disease and those who are free of the disease. The rows distinguish between exposure to an element, factor, or environmental insult. This simple table can be read from top to bottom or from left to right. Case–control studies typically view two groups in the population – an affected group (with the disease) and a comparable group (free of disease). A retrospective study looks back to identify differences in the experiences of the two groups. Cohort studies follow two groups: one group of people exposed to say, for example, cigarette smoke, and a similar group who are not exposed to smoke.

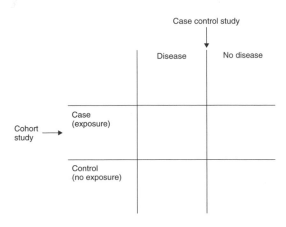

Figure 7.2 Case control and cohort study 2 × 2 model

Prospective cohort studies are more powerful than case–control studies. Issues relating to time, e.g. 'when did it begin?' and 'when does it stop?' can be established in a prospective study, and confounders (contextual factors that do not have a direct bearing on outcomes) are more easily controlled for. However, prospective studies are more costly, and there is a greater chance of losing subjects to follow-up based on the long time period over which cohorts are typically followed (see 'What's the evidence?' for an example).

What's the evidence?

Hannaford and colleagues ('Mortality among contraceptive pill users: cohort evidence from Royal College of General Practitioners' Oral Contraception Study', *BMJ* 2010; 340: c927) reported on a cohort study, which examines if the mortality risk among women who have used oral contraceptives differs from that of women who have never used the contraceptive pill. The study started in 1968 and involved more than 46,000 women, observed for up to 39 years. Look up this study to explore its key findings.

Qualitative research studies

While quantitative research is used to test a hypothesis, qualitative research is used for exploration. Qualitative research is used to gain insight into people's attitudes, behaviours, value systems, concerns, motivations, aspirations, culture or lifestyles. Qualitative research seeks out the 'why', the meaning, and not the 'how' of its topic through the collection and analysis of semi- or unstructured information. Focus groups, in-depth interviews, content analysis, ethnography, evaluation and semiotics are among the many approaches that are used in qualitative research.

Qualitative research is often used to explore a new phenomenon, and the results from such exploratory qualitative studies can be used to inform the planning and design of quantitative studies (e.g. an RCT). It is also common to carry out qualitative work alongside an RCT to explore why an intervention worked, or did not work: interviews with study participants may, for example, indicate that they found the drug regimen under study too onerous and hence did not comply with it as instructed.

Because of the type of research questions under investigation in qualitative research studies, sample sizes are usually quite small but selected because they have certain characteristics (e.g. teenagers with asthma who have had a recent admission to hospital). However, analysis of relatively unstructured, 'wordy' data is time-consuming and just as skilled as 'number-crunching' quantitative data. Many qualitative methods require researchers to carefully code data and discern and document themes consistently and reliably.

We have introduced a few key research methods here, to illustrate how different study designs are appropriate to different research questions. We now look at how to sift through, or critically appraise, studies and papers so you can apply findings from the literature to answer questions raised by specific clinical problems.

Applying scientific method and approaches

Critical appraisal

We are faced with an enormous amount of published scientific work. The search for information about drug X would have revealed a lot of research studies all of potential interest.

Your task as a reader is to make an assessment of the reliability and validity of research papers. In simple terms, the reliability is the repeatability of a study (i.e. if you repeated this study in broadly the same terms, it would produce broadly the same results). The validity is a more complex construct about the strength of the conclusions of the study – it encompasses both the relationship between the intervention and the outcome, and also the generalisability of the findings.

The process of assessing research studies is termed critical appraisal. The purpose of critical appraisal is not to destroy a piece of work, or to show the cleverness of the critic. There is always something that can be criticised in a study. Often, and especially in studies of health and of health services, investigators have carried out the best study possible in the (often-difficult) circumstances. The challenge is to establish what useful lessons can be learned from a study, despite any flaw in the study.

How to read a paper critically

In critical appraisal, we take an article that caught our eye or one that we have found through a database search and read it to determine whether it might influence our practice one way or another.

Firstly, it is useful to know a little about how articles are typically presented. Research studies are written using the *IMRaD* convention: the *introduction* gives the background and describes other work in this field and why this study is needed; the *methods* outline how, when, and where the study was done, what was measured and by whom; the *results* describe what was found; the *discussion* reviews what the results mean for individuals, clinical practice, and population health, and compares findings with other studies; and the *conclusion* covers implications for further research. The studies will have a title, a summary or abstract, various tables and figures, and a list of references, all of which can be useful in critical appraisal.

Scanning original studies can be useful: is the title interesting or useful? Does the summary present some potentially useful results? If the setting of the study is comparable to where you work, would these results apply in your population? However, while scanning is useful, we do need to be more rigorous and structured in our appraisal. To illustrate critical appraisal in action, we look at how to appraise an RCT.

There are three broad areas to consider (See Guyatt *et al.*, 1993a, 1993b):
Is the trial valid?

- Can I 'trust' the results? (The results might suggest that ten times more people get better on the new drug than the existing one, but how do I know that this is really the case? The real test of validity is in the nature and trustworthiness of the methods.)

What are the results?

- Am I impressed by the size or scale of the results with the particular treatment being tested?

Will the results help locally?

- Can I use this treatment with my patient(s)?

ACTIVITY 7.3

Apply these ten questions that may be used for critical appraisal of an RCT to a recent RCT published in a reputable medical journal (try the *BMJ*, *Thorax* or *The Lancet*).

- Did the study ask a clearly focussed question?
- Was the study an RCT and was it appropriately so?
- Were participants appropriately allocated to intervention and control groups?
- Were participants, staff, and study personnel blind to participants' study groups?
- Were all the participants who entered the trial accounted for at its conclusion?
- Were participants in all groups followed up and data collected in the same way?
- Did the study have enough participants to minimise the play of chance?
- How are the results presented (e.g. intention to treat analysis) and what are the main results?
- How precise are the results?
- Were all important outcomes considered and can the results be applied to your local population?

(Critical Appraisal Skills Programme. Appraisal tools. Oxford, UK,
www.phru.nhs.uk/casp/rcts.htm)

The Critical Appraisal Skills Programme (CASP, **www.caspinternational. org**) has produced appraisal checklists to assess the applicability, reliability and validity of published research. CASP has developed appraisal tools, or checklists, to assess many different types of research studies including RCTs, cohort and case control studies, and qualitative research. These tools are extremely useful.

Hierarchies of evidence

There are several hierarchies of evidence based on the powerfulness of the research design in its ability to answer research questions on the effectiveness of interventions. The hierarchy provides a framework for ranking evidence and indicates which type of studies carry most weight. The pyramid shape is used to illustrate the increasing risk of bias inherent in study designs as one goes down the pyramid.

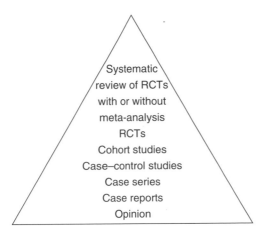

Figure 7.3 Hierarchy of evidence for questions about the effectiveness of an intervention or treatment.

Source: Craig and Smyth, 2002. Reproduced with permission © Elsevier.

At the top are systematic reviews which combine individual research studies by the research topic, the subjects and the generalised measurable outcomes (see later in this chapter for further discussion of systematic reviews). Large quantities of information are put into a manageable form. Systematic reviews identify and explain inconsistencies, and have cut the lag between theory and practice in a number of areas of practice. A single case study is always going to be less persuasive than a collection of studies, if they are available and/or comparable.

Research synthesis

There are literally tens of thousands of research papers published every year in the medical literature. For the majority of doctors who serve populations in the NHS it is just not possible to keep abreast of the research output that relates to clinical practice. Synthesising research output is a real skill and creating a repository of the accumulated findings of medical research is a vital resource. Why is this? Decisions are most beneficial when informed by a consideration of all the available evidence rather than just an individual study.

The greatest challenge to the process of systematic review is heterogeneity as the treatment, patients and outcomes must be comparable between the various studies.

The study design, study quality, and characteristics of the individuals in each study, and the outcomes that are measured are all compared.

There are institutions, networks of academics, and professional organisations that sift through research, appraising individual research studies and creating searchable databases of credible outcomes from research studies. The most useful single source of systematic reviews is the Cochrane Collaboration, which produces systematic reviews of healthcare interventions, known as Cochrane Reviews, which are published online in the Cochrane Library (**www.thecochraneli-brary.com**). Cochrane Reviews are often used as the basis of clinical guideline recommendations.

Clinical guidelines

There are a number of organisations whose role is to review the available evidence and advise clinicians on best practice. For example, the National Institute for Health and Clinical Excellence (NICE, **www.nice.org.uk**) and the Scottish Intercollegiate Guidelines Network (SIGN, **www.sign.ac.uk**) produce clinical guidelines and guidance for the NHS. See Chapter 5 for more discussion of clinical guidelines in the context of clinical effectiveness and best practice.

Clinical research and ethics

Research on human subjects is a worthy means of generating valuable information about life-saving techniques and quality of life enhancing treatments. However, research involving experiments on human subjects is burdened with a history of abuse such as Nazi research and the Tuskegee Syphilis trials. As a consequence, careful guidelines and legislation have been designed to protect individuals who participate in human research trials.

The National Research Ethics Service (NRES) safeguards the dignity and welfare of people participating in research in the NHS, and enables research that benefits individuals and society.

Potential research participants at NHS organisations in the UK will come under the protection of the local Research Ethics Committee (REC). RECs scrutinise proposals to ensure that these standards are maintained in all experimentation even with minimal risk and interference. REC is entirely independent of the researcher and the organisations funding and hosting the research.

The members of a REC are specially trained in research ethics and often have the sort of experience which will be useful in scrutinising the ethical aspects of a research proposal. Members include patients, members of the public, nurses, GPs, hospital doctors, statisticians, pharmacists and academics, as well as people with specific expertise gained through a legal, philosophical or theological background.

ACTIVITY 7.4

The National Research Ethics Service (NRES, **www.nres.nhs.uk**) provides full guidance on whether a research project requires review by an NHS Research Ethics Committee, on all tasks involved in taking a project through the process, as well as providing online resources relevant to each stage of the process (e.g. example of a participant consent form). Go to the NRES website. You will see that the website provides much guidance not just on how to apply for ethics review, but also how to complete or create the required documentation. For example, look up the guidance on Patient Information Sheets and Consent Forms.

Although review by a Local Research Ethics Committee (LREC) is not a legal obligation, not seeking approval from an LREC will negatively affect the decisions of grant-funding bodies and make it very unlikely that results will be published in peer-reviewed academic journals. Some study populations do not come under the remit of LREC, specifically those involving undergraduate students. If the study involves students, the source of review is usually a university internal ethics committee.

In reviewing each research proposal submitted, the ethics committee must consider the following:

1. The scientific merit of the proposal.

2. Whether the participant's health may benefit from, or be affected by, the research.

3. Hazards to the participant and whether there are facilities to deal with hazards.

4. The degree of discomfort and distress to the participant.

5. Whether the investigator is adequately qualified and experienced (a CV is submitted with the application).

6. Whether there is any financial or other reward to the doctors, researchers or participants.

7. The need to ensure an adequate consent (see later for discussion of informed consent) has been obtained from the participant.

8. Whether an appropriate information sheet for the subject has been prepared (Participant Information Sheet, the 'PIS').

9. Adequate reparation if the participant is harmed as a direct result of the research (indemnity arrangements).

10. To protect children from harm, they may be included only if no valid alternative exists.

11. Recognition that incompetent patients cannot consent to participate in research, nor can proxy consent be given on their behalf, unless the research is of therapeutic value to the subject. In the case of children they may consent if

they demonstrate Gillick competence, i.e. understanding of the possible risks and effects of the treatment. There are RECs that deal specifically with research projects proposing to involve adults with incapacities.

Informed consent

You may be familiar with the key elements of informed consent in clinical practice. Informed consent is relevant to all healthcare decisions because it protects the rights of individual persons involved in treatment, diagnosis, management and research. All potential research subjects must give voluntary, informed consent in advance of any treatment. Every research project must provide adequate information to potential participants in order to protect their autonomy.

A research study can last a year or more and there might be different phases in a study. It might therefore be necessary to return to the consent process during the study. Implicit in the consent process is the possibility of refusal on the part of the research subjects, and this can be exercised at any point in a study.

Informed consent has several components (see Baum, 1986):

- Information must be presented in a way that can be processed by potential participants and indeed by participants during a study. The information must be imparted by people who have knowledge of the study.

- Understanding by participants must be checked by the research organisers. This can be checked by asking participants to repeat back what they understand the study to be about and what is expected of them.

- Participants must be competent to consent for themselves.

Informed consent for research is very much the same as consent for treatment.

Clinical audit

Audit is a quality improvement process that seeks to improve patient care and outcomes by measuring these against explicit criteria and then through implementing changes. The changes to structures, processes and outcomes are monitored and re-audited over time (see Chapter 5 for a description of the clinical audit process). Audit is a statutory requirement and is a part of the accreditation of doctors, general practices and hospitals.

The idea for an audit may come from a recent research study, a new clinical guideline, a significant event in practice or a notion that someone has about a particular aspect of patient care. For example, a student on a GP placement might see a patient recently discharged from hospital. The patient hands over the discharge sheet, which has spaces for the reason for admission, the drugs on discharge and plans for follow-up. In this particular case, the student notices that the discharge sheet does not record the reason for admission or the diagnosis, which is frustrating since the patient does not understand what they were told. The student decides to audit whether discharge documentation for other patients is completed.

Audit is about benchmarking care against pre-determined standards. In contrast, research is about discovering what the right thing to do is (new knowledge). However, sometimes it can be difficult to decide whether something is research or audit. The National Research Ethics Service provides guidance on how to distinguish between research and audit.

Criteria for audit should derive from good quality evidence. The criteria should relate to important aspects of care that have an influence on outcome (e.g. it may be critical to know of certain diagnoses and of essential follow-up management), and the criteria should be measurable. In the example of discharge sheets above, it is possible to define/measure whether a space in a pro-forma is left blank. For other audit topics, evidence-based guidelines can be a good source of information for selecting criteria.

Setting the standards for audit can be challenging and it is important not to set these too low or too high. It is tempting to state that it is sufficiently important that discharge information is provided that the standard should be 100 per cent. In reality, some information may be missing from the discharge documentation because it was only partially completed when the doctor was called away urgently. The nurses, not wanting to keep a patient back from going home, and certainly not aware that the doctor intended to return to the discharge sheet, gave the patient the form to leave. Taking account of all sorts of instances you might wish to set your target at 75 per cent.

Measuring the level of performance

It is often necessary to sample patient case notes though this may be determined by the purpose of the audit. There may be too many notes (or records) to work through and a '25 per cent sample' or the selection of 'every fifth consecutive patient attending' or 'every fifth patient from the alphabetical database' will have to be agreed. This will depend on whether paper or electronic records are used. If the audit is to identify individual patients from a search of an electronic record system then the records of the entire population of patients is searched. The audit topic often defines the population by age range, gender, disease, investigation or event.

The results of audit are a series of numbers and percentages. Processes and structures are reviewed to ensure that patients leave hospital with copies of relevant and important information. Such changes to processes and practice will improve patient care. It may be difficult to do locally if there are several hospitals.

Audit is included in learning portfolios for doctors and is currently included in appraisal. It is recognised that audit can demonstrate improvements in patient care.

Adverse incidents or 'significant events'

Audit is one tool for improving patient care. Another element of continuous professional development and learning for doctors is reflection on reports of things that have gone particularly well or badly. These are often termed 'significant events' or 'thought-provoking events'. In order to learn from failures, near misses and successes we have to find ways to analyse the events.

NHS errors can have dire consequences for patients and staff, and for wider society. These errors are sometimes blunders, lapses or procedural violations and often imply the blame of individuals. Commonly errors are caused by system failures in staffing, training, maintenance, prioritisation and planning.

In the NHS in England and Wales (for which data is currently available):

- it is estimated that 850,000 adverse events and errors occur every year affecting 1 in 10 hospital admissions;

- one third of adverse incidents lead to patient disability or death;

- adverse events cost approximately £2 billion a year in hospital stays alone;

- clinical negligence claims cost the NHS >£500 milion a year;

- medication errors account for 25 per cent of all events.

Perhaps the most worrying fact is that time and again it is shown how the NHS fails to share opportunities to learn from mistakes and the same devastating mistakes happen over the country. (Note that the UK NHS is by no means unique in terms of this.)

ACTIVITY 7.5

In 2000, the Department of Health (**www.dh.gov.uk**) produced the document 'An organisation with a memory'. This document outlines the potential for learning from things that go wrong in the NHS. The NHS is a huge organisation and the document highlights the very real tragedies (see Chapter 2: Case studies) that are repeated if the NHS does not have a mechanism to share the learning from adverse events.

Taking one of the case studies, consider the events that led to the tragic outcomes, and (in the light of your own experience) consider ways to reduce the likelihood of such events being repeated.

The National Patient Safety Agency (NPSA) (**www.npsa.nhs.uk**) helped the NHS learn from things that went wrong and developed solutions to prevent harm. It worked to foster a culture where errors could be investigated and innovative solutions developed by collecting and analysing information from staff and patients via a national reporting and learning system and other sources. The NPSA website had exemplar tools to download and use in order to analyse adverse incidents in practice.

Reflective practice

Reflection has been mentioned earlier, in relation to learning from adverse events or critical incidents. Reflection is a skill, an attitude, and a mental process that involves thinking. To describe someone as reflective is to describe the habit of consideration and analysis of the why, how and what-ifs of situations. Reflection is about standing in a different place and seeing things from a different perspective, and ultimately doing things differently, for example asking: *why do I do things the way I do?*, and *why do I think this?* It can be particularly useful to reflect on your own values, feelings, thinking and actions, as well as the context of a situation.

Schön (1983) described two types of reflection:

- Reflection-on-action

- Reflection-in-action

Reflection-in-action is reflection that takes place in real time. This is learning 'on the go' by being aware of what we do and how we do what we do. Reflection-on-action usually takes place after an event, or may focus specifically on a thought-provoking event. We commonly think back on what we have done, seen or experienced.

In thinking of situations and people we encounter in our ordinary and professional lives, we consider our feelings and values, the context, and also the codes of practice that underpin our behaviour and attitudes. Students and doctors must learn about themselves before they can confront their biases and prejudices that conflict with patient's values and beliefs, and the profession of medicine.

Most reflection is done in our heads and never written down. One good habit to develop is to keep a reflective journal. In the journal you might record significant things that have happened, your own long- and short-term goals and how these change, your thoughts and emotions about events, and new skills, knowledge and competencies. There are also tools to guide reflective thinking, such as Gibbs' reflective cycle (see Figure 7.4), which is used widely in healthcare education.

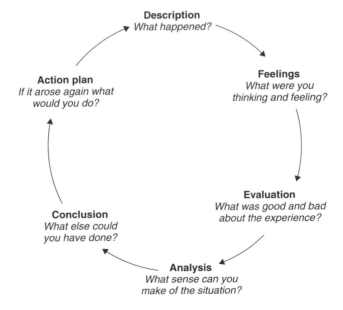

Figure 7.4 Gibbs' (1988) reflective cycle.

Source: Gibbs, G (1988) *Learning by Doing: A Guide to Teaching and Learning Methods*. Further Education Unit. Oxford Polytechnic: Oxford. Reproduced with permission.

Gibbs' reflective cycle can be really useful in making you think through all the phases of an experience or activity. However, if you get frustrated when using a reflective practice tool and cannot record anything at one of the stages in the process, just move on to the next stage.

ACTIVITY 7.6

Select an event that has some meaning to you from your clinical placements. The event might involve a patient you saw in hospital or in the community, and could be a communication issue, whether good or poor. Reflect on this event using Gibbs' cycle. You may find it useful to write down your thoughts about this experience and your reflection on it.

You may have used words such as trust, responsibility, competence, learning, being well, working with uncertainty, and questioning the status quo. Reflecting like this will raise ethical and professional issues that you will certainly come back to time and again.

It is tempting to remember and record only those things that don't go so well. While learning from failure can be valuable you should remember that it is equally valuable to learn from success. It is probably quite important to seek some clarity on why you engage in reflection, and on what you wish to achieve as a result of reflection. Reflection makes a difference to how you feel, think and get things done.

Reflection not only increases one's self-awareness but also can influence competence. In this respect, self-rating of skills can be a useful adjunct to reflection. This is often done using statements such as: *I know this because . . ., I showed this when* . . . against pre-determined criteria. You can also use your own lists. For example, try to come up with a list of six or so ways to describe the kind of doctor you aspire to be, such as 'good listener'. List these attributes and skills, then rate yourself against them. Re-visit this table later in the year and rate yourself again and reflect on your development.

Case study

As you know, Bill has COPD.

COPD management is described in national and international evidence-based guidelines (e.g. **http://guidance.nice.org.uk/CG101**).

NICE grades evidence (critically appraises individual research studies) using a systematic review process which involves assessing the quality of the methods and methodology used in individual studies using an algorithm and checklists. The strength of each recommendation is determined by the robustness of the underlying evidence. The top level of evidence is 1a (high-quality meta-analyses, systematic reviews of RCTs, or RCTs with a very low risk of bias) to 4 (expert opinion, formal consensus), which is translated into grading of recommendations in the format of A–D (where A is based on hierarchy 1 evidence). Influenza vaccinations are recommended in the treatment of COPD (evidence grade IIa).

Bill's GP realised that Bill had not received his flu jab in the previous few years. It was not clear from the records whether or not this had been offered, but refused by Bill, or not offered. She decided to carry out an audit of patient files to investigate whether or not the records recorded a reason for no flu jab. This identified that records were not sufficiently comprehensive, so the practice instigated a new recording system. Not offering a flu jab to a patient with COPD has implications not just in terms of best practice but also in terms of practice payments so the standard for recording was set at 100 per cent, to be reviewed 12 months later. Bill was recalled by the practice for his jab, and attended for this quite willingly – he had wondered why it had not been offered again but did not like to raise this with his GP as he does not like to raise too many issues in his appointments (he is aware that appointment time is limited).

Chapter summary

This chapter provides an introduction to sources of evidence such as books, journal articles and research studies. We have provided a basic introduction to research methods and design, and to tools to use in your clinical practice such as critical appraisal, audit and reflection. These are complex subjects so we have provided a number of links to useful sources of information and further reading so you can explore these topics in more depth in your own time.

GOING FURTHER

Bowling, A (2009) *Research Methods in Health: Investigating Health and Health Services.* Open University Press.
This handbook helps researchers to plan, carry out, and analyse health research, and evaluate the quality of research studies.

Declaration of Helsinki. World Medical Association Declaration of Helsinki: Recommendations Guiding Medical Doctors in Biomedical Research Involving Human Subjects.
The statement of ethical principles for medical research involving human subjects.

Greenhalgh, T (2010) *How To Read a Paper: The Basics of Evidence-Based Medicine*, 4th edition. Wiley-Blackwell.
A really accessible and useful book with lots of helpful hints and tips for what to look for when appraising a paper.

Harris, M and Taylor, G (2008) *Medical Statistics Made Easy*. Scion Publishing.
Does what it says on the front cover!

chapter 8

Activity Limitation and Disability

*Philip Cotton, Jim McKillop and
Jennifer Cleland*

Achieving your medical degree

This chapter will help you to meet the following requirements of *Tomorrow's Doctors*
(2009).

9 Apply psychological principles, method and knowledge to medical practice.

   (b) Discuss psychological concepts of health, illness and disease.
   (c) Apply theoretical frameworks of psychology to explain the varied responses
        of individuals, groups and societies to disease.
   (d) Explain psychological factors that contribute to illness, the course of the
        disease and the success of treatment.
   (f) Discuss adaptation to major life changes, such as bereavement; compar-
        ing and contrasting the abnormal adjustments that might occur in these
        situations.

10 Apply social science principles, method and knowledge to medical practice.

   (b) Discuss sociological concepts of health, illness and disease.
   (c) Apply theoretical frameworks of sociology to explain the varied responses
        of individuals, groups and societies to disease.
   (d) Explain sociological factors that contribute to illness, the course of the
        disease and the success of treatment – including issues relating to health
        inequalities, the links between occupation and health, and the effects of
        poverty and affluence on health and well-being.

11 Apply to medical practice the principles, method and knowledge of population
    health and the improvement of health and healthcare.

   (d) Discuss the principles underlying the development of health and health
        service policy, including issues relating to health economics and equity, and
        clinical guidelines.
   (f) Evaluate and apply epidemiological data in managing healthcare for the
        individual and the community.
   (j) Discuss from a global perspective the determinants of health and disease
        and variations in healthcare delivery and medical practice.

Introduction

Good Medical Practice (**www.gmc-uk.org/guidance/good_medical_practice. asp**) states that doctors must not unfairly discriminate against patients by allowing their personal views to adversely affect their professional relationship with patients or the treatment they provide or arrange. Good Medical Practice specifies that this includes your views about a patient's age, colour, culture, *disability*, ethnic or national origin, gender, lifestyle, marital or parental status, race, religion or beliefs, sex, sexual orientation, or social or economic status. Additionally, you should challenge colleagues if their behaviour does not comply with this guidance. Be aware of your own attitudes, and prejudices, towards disability and take steps to address these by finding out more about common disabilities.

Disability is a huge topic which encompasses, and illustrates, many of the learning outcomes of *Tomorrow's Doctors*. This chapter provides a framework within which to consider definitions and models of disability, its range, scope for prevention and intervention, attitudes towards disability, and the impact of disability on society and the individual.

ACTIVITY 8.1

Before reading this chapter, stop and think.

What does the term 'disability' mean to you?

Disability is a descriptive term. The Disability Discrimination Act (1995) defines a person with disabilities as one *with physical, sensory or mental impairment which has a substantial, adverse and long term (>12 months) effect on 'normal' day to day activities.* The Act was updated in 2010 when the Equality Act became law (**www.equalities.**

gov.uk/equality_act_2010.aspx). Disability is one of the protected characteristics in the new legislation. Other protected characteristics include age, race and
sexual orientation. Under the Equality Act, a person has a disability if they have a
mental or physical impairment that has a continuing effect on their ability to perform day-to-day activities.

Impairments can be cognitive or physical under-development, functional limitation or absence, which can be due to many different conditions and influences
including genetic and chromosomal disorders, accidents and chronic diseases. Some
disabilities may be present from birth, for instance cerebral palsy, and may affect
an individual throughout their lifetime whereas other disabilities might be due to
work-related injuries, such as loss of a finger or sight, or the onset of progressive (e.g.
multiple sclerosis) or chronic diseases (e.g. rheumatoid arthritis) in middle age. The
impacts of a disability on the person and their family will, in part, depend on the
stage of life in which it occurs.

The World Health Organization (WHO, 2008a) estimates that about 650 million people live with disabilities of various types (see Figure 8.1), and the number
is increasing due to the rise of injuries from car crashes, falls and violence, and
chronic diseases associated with ageing. Figure 8.1 shows that disability prevalence
raises sharply with age. Of this total, 80 per cent live in low-income countries; most
are poor and have limited or no access to basic services, including rehabilitation
facilities. Although older people make up a great proportion of the population in
high-income counties they have lower levels of disability than their counterparts in
low- and middle-income countries. Disability is also more common among children
in low- and middle-income countries.

These facts are not independent of each other, but all indicate that the risk of
becoming disabled has a strong correlation with the individual's socio-economic
status. In other words, those who are already disadvantaged are at significantly
greater risk of becoming disabled. There are strong associations between being poor,

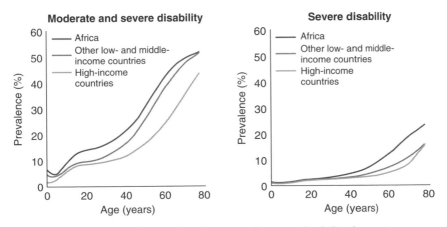

Figure 8.1 Estimated prevalence of moderate and severe disability by region, sex and
age, global burden of disease estimates for 2004. From **www.who.int/healthinfo/
global_burden_disease/2004_report_update/en/index.html** p. 33.

UK facts and figures

The UK governmental Office for Disability Issues (**http://odi.dwp.gov.uk/disability-statistics-and-research**) provides up-to-date and comprehensive data on disability in the UK. Here are some basic facts and figures in 2011 relating to people with a registered disability:

- There are over 10 million people with a limiting long-term illness, impairment or disability in the UK.
- The prevalence of disability rises with age. Around one in 20 children have disabilities, compared to around one in seven working-age adults and almost one in two people over state-pension age.
- A substantially higher proportion of individuals who live in families with disabled members live in poverty, compared to individuals who live in families where no one has a disability.
- The employment rates of people with disabilities are around 48 per cent, compared with around 78 per cent of non-disabled people.
- People with disabilities are around twice as likely not to hold any qualifications compared to non-disabled people, and around half as likely to hold a degree-level qualification.
- People with disabilities are significantly more likely to experience unfair treatment at work than non-disabled people.
- Around a third of people with disabilities experience difficulties related to their impairment in accessing public, commercial and leisure goods and services.

being out of work, having low educational qualifications and the risk of developing a long-term health problem or impairment. Furthermore, people who experience an unexpected deterioration in their health, or who have an accident, have larger falls in household income than those whose condition develops gradually. Disability is not a minor issue to be ignored. As a practising doctor you will encounter people with various forms of disability throughout your working life.

Models of disability

There are several different models of disability, each of which has contributed to a broader understanding of disability and activity limitation. We will discuss each of these in turn.

Medical model

This model regards disability as intrinsic to the individual, a direct consequence of an underlying disease or disorder. From this perspective, reductions in disability can only be achieved through the amelioration of underlying pathology. Medical intervention is therefore viewed as the means to restore 'normality'.

The model does not take into account that pathology is a poor predictor of disability. For example, with reference to our running COPD case study, lung function does not predict dyspnoea: social and psychological factors play a large role in an individual's perception of breathlessness. Another difficulty with the medical model of disability is that its person-centred focus encourages stigmatisation and negative labelling. Think of attitudes towards people with epilepsy, or people who have been patients in a psychiatric hospital, or towards those with smoking-related diseases or obesity. Research shows that stigmatisation and negative labelling affect the behaviour of the individual with the disability, the social responses of other people to the difference, and may also play some part in medical decision-making. For example, in the past, people with epilepsy, cerebral palsy or low ability were often institutionalised as being dangerous to the public.

People with physical disabilities have been segregated in the past by ordinances such as Chicago's 'ugly law', which prohibited 'diseased, maimed, mutilated . . . or deformed' persons from appearing in public. Eugenicists lobbied for sterilisation of people with various disabilities.

Social model

This model places the disability outside the individual. The focus is socio-cultural. The model focusses on the social and physical environment that causes problems for people with disability. In other words, people are limited not by their medical condition per se but the behaviour of others towards them and by environmental barriers such as inaccessible buildings. Attitudes in the workplace are also important under this model – people with a disability are more likely to be out of work. It becomes the duty of society to remove barriers to participation and to remove the resulting discrimination. The underpinning legislation, such as the Disability Discrimination Act and Equality Act, is designed to help remove such barriers and address socio-cultural barriers for people with disabilities.

This social model helps us to determine what we can do to influence ways to reduce limitations people may experience. Provision of designated car parking spaces, wheelchair access to public buildings, guide dogs, the provision of utility bills in Braille, loop systems on telephones and museum audio guides are all attempts to overcome problems of access for individuals with various impairments. Cultural barriers may, however, be more difficult to address than environmental ones. Different cultures have different attitudes towards disability. The definitions of disability used in this chapter are Western and describe a series of values, judgements and attitudes that are part of our culture; disability is not viewed in the same terms or explained in the same way in other cultures. Indeed many languages do not have a word for 'disability'. Even within the same culture there may be conflicting beliefs about disability, for example, that a particular disability might result from an 'accident', a genetic disorder, an act of judgement that can be a punishment or a blessing, or from an infection.

Disability is often explained in terms of 'blame', irrespective of whether religious or medical explanations dominate. Blame is often directed towards women (i.e. a child has a disability because their mother has failed in some way) or other minority groups, for example a man is HIV-positive because he is gay. In many cultures, having a disability is attributed to having sinned or offended the spirits. This might have occurred through sins committed by ancestors or by the person with the disability themselves in this or a previous life. What is generally understood about the relationship between culture and disability is based predominantly in the cultures of the Western world. This is despite the fact that about 80 per cent of all individuals with disability live in developing countries.

How disability is legally defined influences how people with disability are treated within a society. In the past, the dominant approach was paternalistic (see Chapter 1). However, in developed countries, people with disability have lobbied hard to have their voices heard and to bring about change in societal structures, legislative and policy reform, the reorganisation of the disability sector, and improvements in community attitudes and awareness of disability. The word deaf with a lower case 'd' describes the physical impairment while Deaf with a capital 'D' describes the culture which has existed for many years. People born deaf belong to a world that has its own language form, culture and arts, and history. 'Deaf' people perceive themselves as culturally deaf and attend schools for the deaf and initiatives for the deaf.

Psychological model

The psychological model of disability emphasises that activities performed by someone with a health condition are influenced by the same psychological processes that affect the performance of these behaviours by non-disabled people. These include motivation, mood disorders (depression, anxiety) and self-efficacy (see also Chapter 3). They may also include factors such as upbringing (which contributes to the development of resilience, coping and self-motivation (see also Chapter 2). Two people with the same medical condition living in the same social and environmental situation may have very different activity limitations due to their cognitions, emotions and coping strategies. For example, stroke patients with a stronger belief that they can influence their recovery do more activity than those with less belief in personal control (Johnston et al., 2005). Indeed, research has repeatedly shown that improved psychological states influence recovery from activity limitations. How people cope with disability can also be influenced by the reactions of their family and friends, and the professionals with whom they are in contact.

As well as taking into account psycho-emotional dimensions of disability, the psychological model acknowledges the lived experience of disability. This includes how one is treated by others and one's self-image (e.g. the change from being a healthy person to a person with a disability in those who develop limitations). The lived experience of disability may also include social and economic marginalisation, uncertainty and fear about future well-being, and feelings of powerlessness. Those living with a disability tend to have poorer psycho-emotional well-being, and this is related not just to psychological factors but also to social attitudes towards disability (see earlier).

These models can help us to understand and empathise with a person who has a disability. However, working in teams within the health service to meet the needs of all people who become patients requires the use of a common vocabulary rather than separate models. This has significance when legislating for society and when planning for adaptations for individuals. This common model is provided by the International Classification of Functions (ICF) Framework published by the World Health Organization (WHO) in 2001 (see Figure 8.2). The ICF is a classification of health and health-related domains. These domains are classified from body, individual and societal perspectives by means of two lists: a list of body functions and structure, and a list of domains of activity and participation. These classifiers are available on the WHO ICF website (**www.who.int/classifications/icf/en**). Since an individual's functioning and disability occurs in a context, the ICF also includes a list of environmental factors.

You can see that the ICF incorporates aspects of the medical, social and psychological models of disability.

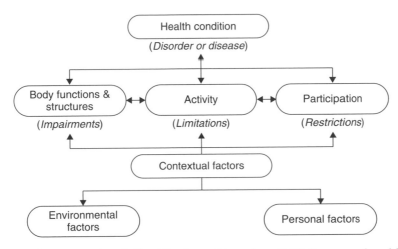

Figure 8.2 The International Classification of Functions (ICF) Framework published by the World Health Organization (WHO).

In the ICF, functioning is considered as the body or body part, the whole person, and the person in their daily life.

For example, for a person with COPD, the lungs are principally affected and restricted lung function can limit physical activity. People with COPD may be limited in the ways that they get around the home and when outside. They may find that some of the activities necessary to look after themselves such as showering, shopping and cleaning are limited. They may also find that they are restricted and can no longer access leisure and social areas because of distance or design. Furthermore, in the ICF the interaction with contextual factors is described as environmental factors and personal factors. For a person with COPD and specifically with shortness of breath on minimal exertion, the physical challenges of negotiating public transport and buildings (environmental factors) may impact on the ability to participate in social and other activities such as going to the bank or shops. Other environmental factors include social attitudes; for example some people may not tolerate others – perhaps with COPD – who cannot keep up in group activities.

People with COPD may have developed a fair degree of resilience and coping strategies (personal factors) that get them through a day of essential activities. The personal factors are influenced by age, gender, profession and other individual attributes, e.g. someone in a respected post in a sedentary job with a lot of administrative support may be in a very different situation from someone with a similar grade of severity of COPD who is in a manual job without support.

The ICF describes a dynamic interaction between domains and factors so that an intervention in one domain affects others. For example, easy access to public buildings or help with self-care.

The ICF acknowledges that every human being can experience a decrement in health and thereby experience some degree of disability. Disability is not something that only happens to a minority of humanity. The ICF thus 'mainstreams' the experience of disability and recognises it as a universal human experience. By shifting the focus from cause to impact, it places all health conditions on an equal footing allowing them to be compared using a common metric – the ruler of health and disability.

As mentioned earlier, attitudes towards disability are critical in determining how people with disability are viewed by society. Unhelpful attitudes may, in part, arise because many people do not have contact with disabled people. A lack of understanding of the nature of disability or of what it is like to live with impairment will influence views of disability, often leading to fear (e.g. becoming disabled is the worst thing that could happen to me). While many medical students will have had contact with disability (their own, that of a family member or friend) and thus may have quite a good understanding of what it is like to live with a disability, others will not. Society as a whole is exposed to negative views and misperceptions of disability, the latter being commonly fostered by the mass media, and these can lead to discrimination.

ACTIVITY 8.2

Seven types of discrimination are described in the 2010 Equality Act. Search the Equality Act website (**www.equalities.gov.uk/equality_act_2010.aspx**) to find the definitions of each of the following terms. Before you do, however, how many of the definitions do you know?

- Direct discrimination
- Associative discrimination
- Indirect discrimination
- Harassment
- Harassment by a third party
- Victimisation
- Discrimination by perception

Understanding discrimination will help you avoid being discriminatory in your medical practice.

For example, the language surrounding disability within mainstream media is often very negative (e.g. 'cripple'), particularly regarding hidden impairments. If someone with dyslexia is mocked in a newspaper, the consequences might be that people with dyslexia are thought of as 'thick', and other people with dyslexia may not declare their disability for fear of the same treatment. This can lead to lack of support, which can in turn mean they struggle in their job, or their studies, and could potentially lead to low self-esteem and depression. The creation and perpetuation of stigmas (see earlier) creates a vicious cycle where people with hidden impairments isolate themselves through not declaring their impairment. Because they do not declare or discuss their impairment, other people in society don't have an understanding of the reality of the impairment.

As a medical student, you will have opportunities to meet people with a range of disabilities. These will include hidden disabilities (e.g. dyslexia, COPD, epilepsy), to those which are very obvious (e.g. the loss of a limb from an accident or peripheral neuropathy, Down syndrome, a progressive, degenerative disease requiring wheelchair use, a sensory loss requiring a guide dog or hearing aid), to those where impairment fluctuates (e g rheumatoid arthritis where people often report 'good days and bad days') and those which are due to poor outcome of treatment/surgery (e.g. Dumping syndrome in people who have had stomach surgery). Use these opportunities well – find out from the individuals what they find difficult on a day-to-day level, if they have experienced any discrimination or negative attitudes, what would make a difference to their quality of life (see later). We know from our own experience that students who have direct contact with people with disabilities are more likely to use positive words and words associated with the social model of disability when describing personal attributes of people with disability after their course. Increased understanding of disability will help you be a good doctor to your patients.

ACTIVITY 8.3

Consider where disability is taught and assessed in your medical degree curriculum. You may have had tutorials and lectures flagged up as covering the topic of disability. However, think more broadly than this: where have you learned about, or met, people with a disability? Think about your general practice, ward and clinic experiences. With the ICF definition in front of you, consider also your personal experiences and the people you know – would you now consider someone as having a disability who you had not seen as such before reading the ICF?

Assessment of disability

Disability is typically assessed by activities of daily living (ADL) and quality of life (QoL) measures.

ADL measures assess the person's ability to perform everyday self-care or mobility activities. They can be self-reported or observational. The former requires individuals to describe difficult experiences while the latter requires the individual to perform defined activities while an observer notes successes and failure. Both approaches have pluses and minuses. Self-report allows assessment of a wide range of activities, occurring in the home or in other situations, at all times of day and night, and over days, weeks or months. Self-report also allows the individual to highlight activities which are especially important to them (e.g. gardening, walking the dog, reading). Observational methods of assessing ADL are more objective but are restricted to what can be assessed in hospital or during a relatively brief home visit.

The Barthel Index of Activities of Daily Living

The Barthel Index (Mahoney and Barthel, 1965) is commonly used to assess ADL. It consists of 10 items that measure a person's daily functioning. The items include feeding, moving from wheelchair to bed and return, grooming, transferring to and from a toilet, bathing, walking on level surface, going up and down stairs, dressing, continence of bowels and bladder. The assessment can be used to determine a baseline level of functioning and can be used to monitor improvement, or deterioration, in activities of daily living over time. The higher the score the more 'independent' the person.

The Barthel Index tends to be used in hospitals, for people with quite severe disability. There are other ADL measures more commonly used in community settings, or to assess rehabilitation outcomes, and measures designed for specific groups (e.g. stroke patients, children) such as the Functional Motor Test.

Functional capacity is often assessed just as much as incapacity. A person's performance may be influenced by the actual loss of function (such as by physical limitation), restrictions on function (such as advice not to perform certain activities), premature termination of activity and suboptimal performance (possibly limited by pain and fatigue, environment, motivation and attitude). The approach is increasingly to combine the medical, psychological and social models so that, overall, disability is seen to depend not only on bodily or mental impairment but also on performance and behaviour. Thus 'ability' may be set by physiological or pathological limits, whereas actual performance is often set by psychosocial limits including the limits set by the person's specific environment.

Quality of life

Quality of life (QoL), or to be more precise, health-related QoL (HRQoL), includes the physical, functional, social and emotional well-being of an individual. QoL judgements are based on the gap between the real and the ideal, and centre on considering the person's hopes and reality and determining the breadth of the gap between them. The narrower the gap the greater is the quality of life.

HRQoL is a patient-reported outcome usually measured with questionnaires or semi-structured interview schedules (i.e. not just with asking your patient how they feel today!). HRQoL measures allow comparison of patients' functional health status over time and in comparison to other patients, and help doctors understand the outcomes of their interventions.

Some HRQoL measures are unidimensional (i.e. they only measure one thing, such as pain or anxiety). Others are multi-dimensional, covering physical, functional, psychological/emotional and social/occupational aspects of daily living. Tools can also be generic (e.g. the SF-36, Ware and Sherbourne, 1992) or disease-specific HRQoL (e.g. the Asthma Quality of Life Questionnaire, Juniper *et al.*, 1992). Disease-specific instruments are known to be more sensitive to assess changes within patients while generic instruments are less sensitive to assess intra-individual changes, but are specifically designed to detect differences between individuals from a general population (and so can be used to compare QoL across different diseases).

HRQoL assessments are important not just when assessing disability but also to assess treatment benefits. In many situations, for example, when chemotherapy is given for palliation in advanced cancer, QoL is arguably the sole criterion of efficacy. The provision of an artificial limb or prosthesis can make a great difference to QoL in terms of independence and confidence for someone with an amputation.

ACTIVITY 8.4

Quality of life measures are not commonly used in routine clinical practice. Can you think why this may be the case? Consider this question from the point of view of the doctor and the patient.

Compression of morbidity

This theory states that the lifetime burden of illness could be reduced if the onset of chronic illness could be postponed and if this postponement could be greater than increases in life expectancy (Fries, 1980). Good preventive medicine and a healthy lifestyle can postpone disability due to chronic illness, but there comes a stage in every person's life where significant illness-related debility is experienced. As illness progresses, not only do people have to endure many distressing symptoms, they also experience diminished functionality and social isolation. Most become dependent on care provided by close family members. Many people feel that they are burdening their loved ones and this leads to secondary feelings of depression, anxiety and grief.

The compression of morbidity principle states that the objective of increasing life span should be associated at the same time with an increasing quality of life or reduction of disability: there is no point in increasing life span if disability is high and QoL is low. For example, palliative care is concerned with addressing this issue by improving end-of-life care for all patients with major illnesses. Patient-centred evaluation of HRQoL and their views of continued treatment of illness are core to palliative care.

Quality-adjusted life years and resource allocation

HRQoL is also used to determine resource allocation and healthcare policy. All healthcare systems have to confront the economic reality of a finite budget and infinite demands. Utility-based measures, which include QoL measures, are used to generate quality-adjusted life years (QALYs).

Although one treatment might help someone live longer, it might also have serious side effects. For example, it might make them feel sick, put them at risk of other illnesses or leave them permanently disabled. Another treatment might not help someone to live as long, but it may improve their QoL while they are alive, for example, by reducing their pain or disability. The QALY method enables measurement of these factors so that different treatments for the same and different conditions can be compared. A QALY gives an idea of how many extra months or years of life of a reasonable quality a person might gain as a result of treatment – particularly important when considering treatments for chronic conditions.

How a QALY is calculated

The National Institute of Clinical Excellence (NICE) provides a very clear example of how a QALY is calculated on their website: www.nice.org.uk/newsroom/features/measuringeffectivenessandcosteffectivenesstheqaly.jsp.

Patient x has a serious, life-threatening condition.

- If he continues receiving standard treatment he will live for 1 year and his quality of life will be 0.4 (0 or below = worst possible health, 1= best possible health).
- If he receives the new drug he will live for 1 year 3 months (1.25 years), with a quality of life of 0.6.

The new treatment is compared with standard care in terms of the QALYs gained:

- Standard treatment: 1 (year's extra life) x 0.4 = 0.4 QALY
- New treatment: 1.25 (1 year 3 months extra life) x 0.6 = 0.75 QALY

Therefore, the new treatment leads to 0.35 additional QALYs (that is: 0.75 – 0.4 QALY = 0.35 QALYs).

- The cost of the new drug is assumed to be £10,000, but the standard treatment costs £3000.

The difference in treatment costs (£7000) is divided by the QALYs gained (0.35) to calculate the cost per QALY. So the new treatment would cost £20,000 per QALY.

QALYs are utilised by health economists to calculate the cost–utility of different interventions. Each drug is considered on a case-by-case basis.

Policy makers may set certain QALY thresholds. The use of these thresholds by regulatory bodies when making decisions regarding NHS payments for treatments is controversial. Basically, QALYs help decide which healthcare needs will be met by identifying which treatment produces

- the greatest amount of good for,
- the greatest amount of time for and
- the greatest number of people.

At the time of writing, if a treatment costs more than £20,000–30,000 per QALY, then it would probably not be considered cost-effective.

This all sounds very straightforward and reasonable but as with most things in life, QALYs are not infallible. Patients' QALYs are assessed and decisions made on the basis of how well a treatment worked for them. The treatment with the most acceptance can then be applied exclusively. But patients are all unique, so what works for many may not work for the individual. (This is the problem with inductive arguments where particulars are used to imply generals.) Another issue is that the scales used to measure QALYs, while well-designed and robustly tested, tend to be quite value-laden and subjective. For example, they assume that living in a wheelchair is of less value. Finally, resources are finite.

Preventing disability

A brief discussion of approaches to prevent disability or limit the incidence of disability in children and adults is appropriate at this point. The three levels of primary, secondary and tertiary prevention (see Chapter 6) can be used as a framework.

There are interventions and initiatives to reduce, prevent or limit the onset of disabling conditions. Public health initiatives to encourage the use of folic acid before and during early pregnancy reduce the mortality from, and severity and incidence of, spina bifida. Disease prevention interventions such as immunisation programmes, screening health education and promotion (e.g. stop smoking) all limit the prevalence and incidence of disease and subsequent disability in the population. Rheumatoid arthritis can disfigure joints and limit activity. Disease-modifying drugs reduce the effects of the joint destruction with the effect of reducing the resulting disability. Splints and aids can be used to limit the disabling effects of arthritis. Physiotherapists and occupational therapists are among the team that can contribute to the care of people with disabling conditions. Furthermore, rehabilitation limits disability by supporting people to resume an optimal level of functioning after, for example, a stroke. Occupational and environmental medicine initiatives to ensure safe working conditions to limit injury are also pertinent here.

There are several current high-profile media cases which raise issues about assisted suicide, the right to life, and disability (see Case studies below).

Case study 1

Dan James, a 23-year-old who had become paraplegic after a rugby accident, died in the Dignitas clinic in October 2008 after assisted suicide. If he had approached you, as his GP, for advice and help before this event what topics would you have covered with him and what principles would have guided your approach?

Case study 2

You are the GP of Anne who is 25 years old. She has learning difficulties and communication problems. She stays with her mother who has recently been diagnosed as having terminal cancer. Her mother has arranged for Anne to live in a partially supervised flat with four other people with similar impairments. Before moving into the new flat, her mother wishes her to be surgically sterilised. Anne has asked to discuss this with you. What areas should you cover with Anne and what preparations would you make?

Another ethical debate that is relevant to prevention of disability is ante-natal screening. For example, you offer routine ante-natal screening that includes tests for Down's syndrome to a 40-year-old couple. They want to refuse on the grounds that they would not wish further investigations or termination of the pregnancy if the test was positive. They ask for your advice. What would you say?

This is a very typical clinical scenario which involves the 'value of life' debate. There are three aspects to this debate: quality, quantity and sanctity of life. Quality and quantity of life are discussed earlier in this chapter, and the compression of morbidity principle is relevant here: are distressing interventions which do no more than delay death without adding any quality to life or reduction in pain or disability tolerable and acceptable? Where treatment offers 'no chance' of survival other than for a short period of time, do the best interests of the patient focus on the relief of any suffering and a peaceful death?

On the other hand, the sanctity of life refers to the view that all life is worth living under any condition. This view tends to be associated with religious perspectives. It eliminates the justifiability of abortion, euthanasia and rational suicide. The sanctity of life view can be contrasted with the 'quality of life' view that does not recognise an absolute right to life nor a duty to preserve it, but rather judges whether a life is worth preserving (or having in the first place) in terms of its quality.

Both views face inherent difficulties. For those who would place great importance upon quality of life, it is difficult to make decisions on this basis as the quality of life is hard to define and measure (Boddington and Podpadec, 1999). Judgements of what constitutes a life of sufficient quality are notoriously variable. Some people would view life with severe mental or physical impairments as not worth living. However, many severely disabled individuals report that they are content with their lives, which they do not regard as having less value than the lives of others. Thus judgements on the quality of life may reveal prejudices or conclusions based on anxieties or preconceptions. With reference back to the social model of disability, you will remember that disability is at least in part a socially created and conditioned state. The sanctity of life argument, on the other hand, eliminates personal judgement about the value of one's own life (remember abortion, euthanasia and rational suicide are unacceptable under this argument).

Furthermore, both views also face the difficulty of who ought to decide what life is valuable and what is not? Someone external to the patient or family may have a clearer picture of the situation, but may not necessarily be objective (one's own views and experiences, both professional and personal are likely to affect judgement) or may not be able to truly know the best for the individual. On the other hand, leaving decision-making to the individual or family preserves autonomy but those involved may be too subjective and may not be able to make a rational decision.

Implications for medical students and doctors

As a doctor you will be the gatekeeper for many key services and as such will have a 'power relationship' with patients. However, the realisation that often the solution is not 'medical', and an appreciation of what can be achieved through team-working and of the expertise of other healthcare professionals are essential.

Some people become dreadfully self-conscious when in stressful or unfamiliar situations. You may need to modify your particular approach to consulting and examining to take account of a patient's disability. If you experience discomfort in dealing with disability make sure that you don't project this onto the person with the disability.

There is an etiquette that provides some reassurance (**www.scips.worc.ac.uk/ etiquette.html**):

- Don't give assistance before asking first if the person wishes for it.

- Don't be upset if assistance is refused (and don't let this stop you offering assistance in the future).

- Don't be afraid to use figures of speech which refer to the impairment, e.g. *Don't hold your breath!* and *You haven't got a leg to stand on!*

- Don't use disabled as a noun – 'the disabled'.

- Don't use negative language such as handicapped, crippled, deformed, retarded.

- Don't use nouns ending in '. . . ic' which replace the identity of the individual, e.g. a spastic, an epileptic, a diabetic. The message is to acknowledge the disease but to put the person first.

Consider the following: the next time you see a patient with a disability, use patient-centred clinical communication skills including open questions to seek their views of what caused the disability and how they think it will be in the future. Their responses may surprise you. You would then use this information to inform further discussions with the patient.

Consistent with the care you give to all patients, ensure that people with disabilities have adequate information in order to take an informed role in their care and decisions about care. Remember that individuals with impairment will often have a great deal of specialist knowledge so don't assume you know best. As a doctor you may have many questions such as *What can be done to achieve best possible function?* but your starting point is always with your patient. And so your first question is *What does the individual (patient) want?* Disability is not a case of 'a + b = c', rather the impact of a limitation on an individual is down to a complex interaction of individual, societal and medical factors. Disability requires a holistic perspective both in terms of understanding what it is like to live with a disability, and how quality of life could be improved, and in terms of working with other professionals to support people with disability most effectively.

To intervene to support individuals and families where a disability is present requires firstly knowing about the nature of the disability. In other words, a diagnosis and assessment of the disability itself is needed. This seems quite obvious but it is not always a straightforward process, particularly in learning disabilities. It is also difficult to establish a prognosis in many conditions. Of course, diagnosis and prognosis may be influenced by the beliefs and behaviour of the individual (see the psychological model of disability earlier in this chapter), and the views of society towards disability.

Intervention in disability is best supported by multi-professional and multi-agency, e.g. NHS, social work, voluntary sector teams. Teams can provide specialist, appropriate and relevant information and advice regarding the disability and its management, and can act as a point of contact between patients and other health and social care services. They often have information to support people with all aspects of living. They will discuss the impact of the diagnosis and offer practical advice for managing this. This may include an assessment by an occupational therapist, for example, for people who are finding it difficult to manage at home with activities like going up and down stairs, getting to the toilet and using the bath. The occupational therapist can give advice and also suggest equipment to improve independence. This may include equipment to help the individual in the bathroom, toilet or kitchen, bedroom lifting equipment, and home alterations such as ramps, wide doors and improved access to bathing facilities.

Multi-disciplinary team input is discussed further in the running case study at the end of this chapter.

Case study

A few years have passed. Bill's symptoms have worsened. His lung capacity and exercise tolerance are very limited. He is still smoking. He has, however, attended a pulmonary rehabilitation course recently, and this has motivated him to do regular walking and make changes to his diet – and he is also trying – again! – to quit smoking with the help of nicotine replacement patches. He knows a lot more about COPD now, and realises how important it is to avoid exacerbations. This has encouraged him to attend for regular reviews and annual vaccinations, and to contact his GP promptly if he has signs of a chest infection.

Bill is determined to keep working. He is lucky because his job is sedentary, and his employer has been very helpful in making reasonable adjustments to accommodate Bill. For example, he now has a disabled parking space and his office has been moved to the ground floor so he does not need to worry about stairs.

He receives the higher rate of the mobility component of Disability Living Allowance so is eligible for the Blue Badge scheme. The Blue Badge scheme is for people with severe mobility problems. It allows badge holders to park close to where they need to go. Bill is determined to keep getting out and about so this helps. He also books a Shopmobility (**www.shopmobility.org.uk**) scooter when he goes to the local shopping mall with Susan on a Saturday. He finds the specially adapted trolleys at the supermarket useful also.

Bill's home has also been assessed by occupational therapy colleagues. They have advised that he needs a walk-in shower. They are helping him seek funding to help with the cost of adapting the bathroom.

Susan worries that Bill will feel worthless if he is no longer able to support the family financially. However, she is relieved that he is now taking more control of his illness rather than burying his head in the sand. She is helping by making sure they still see friends and family as much as possible so he does not become socially isolated.

Chapter summary

This chapter provides an introduction to some of the current legislation and notions of activity limitation and disability. In considering these domains it is important to be reminded of the cultural and societal influences. The various models of disability give some appreciation of these. It is important to be aware of the current UK legislation reflected in the new Equality Act and in the pre-existing legal framework. As medical students and doctors we must be aware not only of the diagnostic and treatment options for the people we care for but also the communication, ethical and legal facets of their care. Some of these are exemplified in this chapter.

GOING FURTHER

Byron, M, Cockshott, Z, Brownett, H and Ramkalawan, T (2005) What does 'disability' mean for medical students? An exploration of the words medical students associate with the term 'disability'. *Medical Education*, 39: 176–183.
Very pertinent and accessible reading.

Downie, RS and Calman, K (1994) *Healthy Respect*. Oxford: Oxford University Press.
The book offers an introduction to the moral concepts and value of healthcare. It is written by a moral philosopher, a doctor and a nurse and contains questions, cases and exercises.

Miller, S, Ross, S and Cleland, J (2009) Medical students' attitudes towards disability and support for disability in medicine. *Medical Teacher*, 31(6): e272–e277.
This study looks at medical student views of disability at medical school and towards inclusion of disabled medical students and doctors.

Price, R (2003) *A Whole New Life: An Illness and a Healing.* New York: Scribner Book Company.
A memoir of the author's experience of living through the treatment of a tumour that destroyed the nerves in his spine and the use of his legs.

chapter 9

Pulling It All Together
Lindsey Pope and Philip Cotton

Achieving your medical degree

This chapter will help you to meet the requirements of *Tomorrow's Doctors* (2009) as presented under the theme of doctor as a scientist and a scholar.

Previous chapters have focussed on specific outcomes from this theme. This final chapter differs as it takes a more holistic approach, one which uses case studies to illustrate how the outcomes introduced in Chapters 1–8 of this book are applied to clinical medicine.

Chapter overview

We are going to consider:

1. How you apply what you now know in your daily practice.
2. How you and your patient link in to the bigger picture.
3. And provide some tips for when you qualify.

What do we actually mean by 'putting it all together'? Well, essentially this is when you take all the knowledge that you have acquired, and use this, in conjunction with appropriate skills and attitudes, to provide high-quality care to the patient sitting in front of you. Indeed, Good Medical Practice (GMC, 2006, p. 6) states:

> *Good doctors make the care of their patients their first concern: they are competent, keep their knowledge and skills up to date, establish and maintain good relationships with patients and colleagues, are honest and trustworthy, and act with integrity.*

Communication skills are a vehicle for you to use the knowledge that you have acquired, as the patient is the source of some of the key information that you will need. This information may be in the form of answers to questions, presence or absence of clinical signs or test results. Your job is then to process all this information and formulate a provisional diagnosis. From this you can develop a management plan based on recognised best practice. You may not immediately know the correct management but you should know where to go to find it. This may involve asking a senior colleague, looking up the British National Formulary (BNF) or a national guideline or using a trusted resource, e.g. an *Oxford Medical Handbook*. (Obviously, an exception to this would be the management of life-threatening emergencies where you would be expected to initiate immediate management.) In a nutshell, 'putting it all together' is getting on and being the doctor you have been trained to be.

In this chapter we're going to use two examples to demonstrate how as a doctor you may need to 'pull together' bits of information from different sources and also that you may need to consider broader implications than just what applies to the patient sitting in front of you.

The first example is that of a 55-year-old male bus driver who has developed symptoms suggestive of Type II diabetes. This case has a community focus and will consider how we apply theory in practice, e.g. lifestyle change, use of guidelines. It will also look at the impact of a new diagnosis on the patient's daily life including work and consider the importance of patient understanding of disease management and self-care. The second example is that of a 26-year-old female patient post-appendicectomy who develops a wound infection due to MRSA. The care of this patient has a secondary care focus initially but demonstrates the importance of working within systems beyond the immediate doctor–patient relationship. It will also be used to consider strategies for preventative medicine on both a local (hospital) and national scale.

After the examples, we will share some top tips based on our own experience as doctors in training, and as doctors involved in medical education.

To consider the first example (below) we're going to use as a framework the section of *Tomorrow's Doctors 3* entitled 'Doctor as a Practitioner'.

Tomorrow's Doctors 3: The Doctor as a Practitioner. Outcomes 13 and 14

13 The graduate will be able to carry out a consultation with a patient.

  (a) Take and record a patient's medical history, including family and social history, talking to relatives or other carers where appropriate.
  (b) Elicit patients' questions, their understanding of their condition and treatment options, and their views, concerns, values and preferences.
  (c) Perform a full physical examination.
  (d) Perform a mental-state examination.
  (e) Assess a patient's capacity to make a particular decision in accordance with legal requirements and the GMC's guidance.
  (f) Determine the extent to which patients want to be involved in decision-making about their care and treatment.
  (g) Provide explanation, advice, reassurance and support.

14 Diagnose and manage clinical presentations.

  (a) Interpret findings from the history, physical examination and mental-state examination, appreciating the importance of clinical, psychological, spiritual, religious, social and cultural factors.

(b) Make an initial assessment of a patient's problems and a differential diagnosis. Understand the processes by which doctors make and test a differential diagnosis.

(c) Formulate a plan of investigation in partnership with the patient, obtaining informed consent as an essential part of this process.

(d) Interpret the results of investigations, including growth charts, X-rays and the results of the diagnostic procedures.

(e) Synthesise a full assessment of the patient's problems and define the likely diagnosis or diagnoses.

(f) Make clinical judgements and decisions, based on the available evidence, in conjunction with colleagues and as appropriate for the graduate's level of training and experience. This may include situations of uncertainty.

(g) Formulate a plan for treatment, management and discharge, according to established principles and best evidence, in partnership with the patient, their carers, and other health professionals as appropriate. Respond to patients' concerns and preferences, obtain informed consent, and respect the rights of patients to reach decisions with their doctor about their treatment and care and to refuse or limit treatment.

(h) Support patients in caring for themselves.

(i) Identify the signs that suggest children or other vulnerable people may be suffering from abuse or neglect and know what action to take to safeguard their welfare.

(j) Contribute to the care of patients and their families at the end of life, including management of symptoms, practical issues of law and certification, and effective communication and teamworking.

Case study: Just not feeling right

Joe Johnston is a 55-year-old male. He has worked as a bus driver since his late teens. He is very overweight and does not have the healthiest of lifestyles. He is also a smoker (10 cigarettes per day). For several months he has been feeling tired all the time, needs to urinate frequently (polyuria), possibly because he is drinking a lot more than usual. He also has a recurrent mouth infection, which he has been self-treating with an oral rinse bought over-the-counter in his local pharmacy. Needing to go to the loo a lot is quite tricky given his job as he has to adhere to routes and timetables. Also, he has had quite a few days off work without clear reason, 'just not feeling right', and his employer has asked him to see the occupational health nurse because of these absences. Joe is trying not to worry about these symptoms too much. His wife, Karen, has only recently persuaded him to see his GP.

Tomorrow's Doctors outcomes detail specific aspects of the doctor–patient consultation (see above). We go through each of these in turn in reference to Joe.

Take and record a patient's medical history, including family and social history, talking to relatives or other carers where appropriate.

Joe has high blood pressure (hypertension) and high cholesterol. He rarely goes to see his GP as he doesn't like to 'bother' her. However, he does attend when called into the practice for screening or review appointments such as to have his blood pressure recorded. He occasionally takes an antacid for heartburn – he buys this from his local supermarket.

Joe lives at home with his wife Karen who works part-time in the local supermarket. Karen is also overweight and smokes a few cigarettes a day. She has tried to quit in the past but always starts back again as she finds she just gains more weight if she stops completely. His two sons are adults with children of their own. He does not know much about their medical history but they seem healthy enough.

Joe's dad died of a myocardial infarction (MI) at age 60 years. His mum is 76 years old. She has hypertension and was diagnosed with multi-infarct (vascular) dementia several years ago. She manages to stay in her own home with a combination of care from Joe's two younger sisters who live locally and a community care package. Joe and his sisters are worried that another stroke will reduce her independence even further, and she will have to go into a care home. One of Joe's sisters also has hypertension.

Elicit patients' questions, their understanding of their condition and treatment options, and their views, concerns, values and preferences.

You may have heard doctors talking about exploring a patient's 'Ideas, Concerns and Expectations'. This is sometimes abbreviated to ICE. Some doctors think it is sufficient to elicit these pieces of information. The key skill is actually to go on and use this information. This not only helps to address a patient's fears but helps to build on your relationship with them. For example, I (L.P.) once had a young female patient who came to see me with symptoms very suggestive of irritable bowel syndrome (IBS). My main differential diagnosis was that of inflammatory bowel disease. When I asked her if there was anything she was worried that it might be, she told me that she worried that she had ovarian cancer. She had recently read an article in a women's magazine, which outlined what she felt were similar symptoms to her own and was terrified that this was what was wrong. After assessing her fully, I explained to her that I thought she had IBS but I also explained why I did not think that she had ovarian cancer. She was reassured by this.

If you do not elicit underlying worries, the risk is that some patients will go away wondering if you've even considered what they were worried about. Also, they may still be worrying about it!

In Joe's case, he hopes he has something reasonably minor but he has a nagging suspicion that he might have diabetes – he had a colleague who complained of similar symptoms and who was then diagnosed with diabetes. Joe is really worried about this because his colleague had to tell the DVLA (Driving and Vehicle Licensing Agency) about his diabetes and ending up leaving his job because of episodes when he did not feel well when driving (almost certainly due to hypoglycaemia). He thinks that he would find it difficult to get any other work 'at his age', especially as driving a bus is the only job he has done for the past 36 years. He assumes that if he does indeed have diabetes, he will need to inject insulin for the rest of his life and will have to cut out cakes and biscuits.

He is worried that he may lose his job because he has needed time off due to tiredness, he runs late due to having to stop between routes to have frequent 'loo breaks', and if he does have diabetes, will he have to leave his job? Not only does he enjoy his job but he needs the money. He doesn't smoke a lot and he would consider quitting completely. A few men at work have stopped and his grandchildren have nagged him and his wife about smoking as they've been learning about it at school.

A useful question is to consider what it is that Joe wants to achieve. If you can understand where the patient is coming from it makes it much easier to engage in a meaningful and productive discussion about their future management. Basically, he wants to know what's wrong with him. He is fed up of feeling run down. He has eventually made an appointment with his GP.

Perform a full physical examination.

In addition to taking a full history (see earlier), Joe's GP carried out a full physical examination, which identified the following:

- BMI 38

- Pulse 84 bpm regular

- Blood pressure 162/98

She also carried out a blood sugar test (finger-prick test) and a urinalysis to measure the amounts of glucose and protein in Joe's urine. She checked his peripheral pulses, which are present, and for any sign of peripheral neuropathy (e.g. loss of sensation in his feet).

Perform a mental-state examination.

Joe is a bit fed up regarding his recent health and is worried about the possibility of losing his job but he is not clinically depressed.

Assess a patient's capacity to make a particular decision in accordance with legal requirements and the GMC's guidance.

There are no concerns regarding Joe's capacity to make decisions. Useful references are the Mental Capacity Act 2005 (England and Wales) or the Adults with Incapacity (Scotland) Act (2000) if you are unsure.

Determine the extent to which patients want to be involved in decision-making about their care and treatment.

Joe expects that his doctor will advise what is in his best interests. That said, he still wants to know why he is being put on certain medicines and to be involved in choices between treatments if appropriate.

Provide explanation, advice and reassurance and support.

It is important that the suspected diagnosis of Type II diabetes is explained to him and what is involved (e.g. further investigations, see later) in confirming this diagnosis. The difference between Type I and Type II diabetes must be explained. Obviously, Joe needs to be reassured that if he has diabetes, there will be treatment and medication that he can be prescribed to help his symptoms with the aim of getting his blood sugar levels under control. The complications of diabetes (e.g. cardiovascular risk, eye, kidney and nerve damage), and how to prevent them, such as diet, foot care and attending regular screening also should be explained.

His smoking and obesity need to be addressed in a supportive and non-judgemental way. At the end of the day, it is his choice if he wishes not to address these issues but his GP and the wider practice team also need to offer support. Although it would be unusual for a patient not to know the risks of being overweight and smoking, it is still important to discuss these with him. Even if Joe decides he doesn't want to make any lifestyle changes at that point, make sure he realises the door is always open to discuss them in future and re-visit this again with him when you see him in future. He has a lot to cope with his new diagnosis and the worry about his job so it may just need a bit of time for him to get his head around this.

Interpret findings from the history, physical examination and mental-state examination, appreciating the importance of clinical, psychological, spiritual, religious, social and cultural factors.

The GP's history taking and examination suggested that a diagnosis of diabetes should be considered, according to National Institute of Clinical Excellence (NICE) guidelines (**http://guidance.nice.org.uk/CG66**). Joe met the criteria on several counts:

- His urine contained glucose.

- His blood glucose levels were high enough to suggest diabetes.

Make an initial assessment of a patient's problems and a differential diagnosis. Understand the process by which doctors make and test a differential diagnosis.

Review of his notes and a focussed clinical history and examination suggested a diagnosis of diabetes.

Formulate a plan of investigation in partnership with the patient, obtaining informed consent as an essential part of the process.

His GP also asked Joe back to do a fasting plasma glucose (FPG) test. This measures blood glucose in a person who has not eaten anything for at least 8 hours.

Interpret the results of investigations, including the growth charts, X-rays and the results of diagnostic procedures as applicable.

In this case, Joe's fasting glucose level of >11.1 mmol/l, confirmed by repeating the test on another day, means he has diabetes (as per current guidelines).

> **Joe's test results:**
>
> Plasma glucose (non-fasting) 14.3 mmol/l
>
> HBA1C (baseline) 9.8 per cent
>
> CHOLESTEROL AND LIPIDS
>
> Total chol 6.7mmol/l
>
> LDL 5.2mmol/l
>
> HDL 1.2mmol/l
>
> Triglycerides 3.3mmol/l
>
> UREA AND ELECTROLYTES
>
> Sodium 142 mmol/l
>
> Potassium 4.1 mmol/l
>
> Urea 6.7 mmol/l
>
> Creatinine 89 µmol/l
>
> Urinalysis shows microalbuminuria.

As you can see, Joe's results are consistent with Type II diabetes.

Synthesise a full assessment of the patient's problems and define the likely diagnosis or diagnoses.

Joe's GP confirmed with him the diagnosis of diabetes. She realised, from her discussion with Joe on the day he attended to discuss his symptoms, that he had considered this as a possible diagnosis. She was also aware that he was very worried about having to use insulin and the threat this would pose to his job. She also knew Joe and his wife were likely to find lifestyle change (e.g. increasing activity, losing weight) difficult but, on the other hand, they always attended review appointments, and kept appointments, which suggested to her that they might benefit from weight management support from the practice.

Thus, the following problems need to be addressed.

Symptom management: commencement of medication. In this case, given he is overweight but has normal kidney function Joe should be started on metformin. Since he has not been prescribed insulin, Joe does not need to inform the DVLA of his condition, unless he has hypoglycaemic episodes, which would not normally be an issue on metformin.

Preventative care: meal planning, physical activity, smoking cessation and attending regular screening to control and prevent complications (see the Quality Outcomes Framework [QOF] for general practice chronic disease management).

This will involve multi-disciplinary input from the dietician (meal planning), health promotion nurse (smoking cessation) and practice nurse (regular HbA_{1c} blood pressure, etc., screening as per QOF [**www.nice.org.uk/aboutnice/qof/qof.jsp**] guidelines). He would also be offered retinal screening.

Ability to do his job: Optimising his symptom management is clearly a way to mini-mise the impact of his health on his job. If Joe were to lose his job, it would likely have a detrimental impact on both his mental and financial health (Waddell and Burton, 2006). It could affect his confidence as a provider to his family and may impact on his relationship with his wife. It may be appropriate for Joe to speak with his employer to see if his duties can be amended in any way to take into account his physical symptoms (e.g. the need to urinate frequently) until his diabetes is better controlled. Metformin is the first-line drug of treatment for Type II diabetes because it has few adverse side effects and is associated with a low risk of hypoglycaemia (which is par-ticularly important given Joe's job).

Make clinical judgements and decisions, based on the available evidence, in conjunction with colleagues and as appropriate for the graduate's level of training and experience. This may include situations of uncertainty.

In Joe's case, the clinical judgement of his GP was to manage his diabetes in pri-mary care rather than referring him for regular check-ups at the eye clinic. However, his GP may refer Joe to secondary care in the future in a number of circumstances (e.g. if he has an infection, hypoglycaemia, hyperosmolar hyperglycaemic state (HHS), any vascular or renal complications, or cataracts). The aims of treatment would be to get Joe's symptoms under control, by following treatment guidelines, and hence minimise the likelihood of complications occurring.

Formulate a plan for treatment, management and discharge, according to established prin-ciples and best evidence, in partnership with the patient, their carers and other healthcare professionals as appropriate.

This involves responding to patients' concerns and preferences, obtaining informed consent, and respecting the rights of patients to reach decisions with their doctor about their treatment and care and to refuse or limit treatment.

It is useful at this point to stop and consider what you actually want to achieve as a doctor. You should then consider this in light of what you know Joe wants to achieve. By understanding where you are both coming from then the doctor and patient can work together for the benefit of Joe's health. It is crucial to know if there is a mismatch in doctor and patient expectations and to explore this if it exists.

Seek first to understand, then to be understood is one of Stephen Covey's (2004, p. 235) seven habits to develop in order to become a successful person. We also think it's one of the most important messages for any doctor to remember when seeing patients.

What does Joe want to achieve?

- To feel better.

- To be able to do his job.

- Maybe to stop smoking – if the doctor thinks it will help and his wife will support him.

What does the doctor want to achieve?

- Ideally, to get Joe to lose weight, increase his activity levels and stop smoking.

- To help Joe understand what diabetes is and how he can self manage this condition.

- To start Joe on the correct treatment as per recommended guidelines (e.g. metformin).

Often as clinicians we focus on what it is that we do to manage a person's illness. In the example of diabetes, we may focus on what medication we are going to start someone on. This is no use if the person doesn't then take the medication as prescribed, as is often the case. So, how do we best help our patients? Yes, we should practise in line with current recognised best practice (e.g. guidelines). We also need to consider how we can encourage our patient to manage his own illness and to feel involved in improving his own health. For Joe, this may involve having a discussion with him and his wife about their smoking and diet and their impact on his diabetes.

Guidelines and protocols exist for the great majority of common clinical conditions. That said, being a doctor involves more than just identifying where on a flow chart a patient lies and applying it. We have already discussed exploring their ideas, concerns and expectations as a way to improve the shared understanding between a doctor and a patient. We cannot imagine that telling a patient that is says on a flowchart that they are to stop smoking would be very patient-friendly. Once you have considered their case in light of the guideline it is important to then share your proposed plan with the patient and discuss the pros and cons of relevant treatment options. In modern medicine, we use the term patient-centred care to reflect the idea that care is tailored to that individual. This refers not only to their presenting problems but also to their beliefs and preferences. If Joe doesn't wish to modify his diet or attend review appointments at the diabetic clinic at the end of the day that is his choice. It is crucial for the ongoing doctor–patient relationship (see Chapter 1) that his wishes are respected even if we disagree with his choices.

Keeping up to date

As you will have no doubt noticed during your time at medical school, guidelines and protocols are constantly being updated to reflect the most recent evidence available. Therefore it is important as a clinician to consider how you are going to stay up to date. Different people do this in different ways – this may depend on your learning style or more practical issues such as the time and resources you have available to do this. The most important thing is to find a method that works for you and can be tailored to suit your individual learning needs.

Some useful learning methods include the following:

1. Reading journals such as the weekly BMJ, or speciality journal (e.g. monthly BJGP).

2. Online learning – there are many websites which offer a menu of online learning modules from which you can choose (e.g. BMJ learning).

3. Small group learning – problem-based small group learning (PBSG) originated in Canada and provides GPs, medical students and trainees groups with modules specific to every day general practice based around case discussion. Small group learning modules exist in all medical specialties.

4. Educational meetings, conferences and courses – these may be specific to your area of speciality or more general. They give the opportunity to learn from others and share best practice with others.

Team working

The importance of working in partnership with colleagues from medicine and the other health and social care professions cannot be emphasised enough. High-quality long-term care cannot be delivered by one individual working in isolation. In our case, various individuals may be involved in Joe's care over the forthcoming years:

1. Practice nurse – in most GP practices, the practice nurse leads on the majority of chronic disease management.

2. Community-based diabetes nurse specialist – increasing numbers of nurse specialists are working with patients in the community. They are usually attached to the hospital speciality teams and are an important point of contact between primary and secondary care.

3. Diabetes clinic – although at the moment Joe can be managed in the community, if his condition were to deteriorate/complication arise then he may be referred to a endocrinologist in the future.

4. Diabetes rehabilitation team – as yet, in the UK diabetes rehabilitation is not as widespread as rehabilitation for COPD (see case study running through this book) or after cardiovascular events. However, there is some evidence of effectiveness of multi-disciplinary intensive exercise and education programmes for people with diabetes who have self-management difficulties. Think back to Chapter 6 – rehabilitation is tertiary prevention, preventing deterioration.

With different people involved in Joe's care, often based in different sites, effective inter-professional communication is critical. Go to the website of any medical defence union (e.g. MDDUS, MDU, MPS) and you will see from their cases that many of the legal claims brought against doctors focus on poor communication, not poor clinical knowledge or skills. Furthermore, many of these claims are due to breakdowns in communication between different professionals which have led to poor patient care, even the death of patients. Thus, in addition to a shared accountability for the quality of care that Joe receives, and avoiding unnecessary duplication of work and tests, effective communication underpins patient safety.

An important part of effective team working and communication is respect for the importance of others' roles. As a GP in a busy urban practice (PC), if my receptionists don't do their job properly then my world will descend into chaos, and vice versa.

Support patients in caring for themselves

Diabetes UK (**www.diabetes.org.uk**) produces many useful documents to educate and empower patients to do what they can to help manage their own condition. It is important that people feel they are responsible for their own health as 99 per cent of the time healthcare is self-care.

Leaflets may not be everyone's cup of tea and perhaps other patients or carers may benefit from being put in contact with local or national support services. It is your responsibility as a doctor to signpost the patient to support options available and to engage them in discussion about how they can best manage their illness.

In Joe's case, there are various areas that he and his wife can consider to try and improve his health in the long term.

- Stop smoking – both him and his wife.

- Take his medicine the way it has been prescribed and let the doctor or nurse know any difficulties he is having with it (e.g. gastrointestinal side-effects).

- Attend for any reviews at his practice, the eye clinic or the diabetes clinic.

- Go to the hospital or seek medical advice if he has a hypoglycaemic or HKK episode.

- Know how to recognise that his blood glucose is out of control and what to do if that happens.

- Keep well by exercising regularly and eating healthy food.

Identify the signs that suggest children or other vulnerable people may be suffering from abuse or neglect and know what action to take to safeguard their welfare.
      This is not applicable in this case.

Contribute to the care of patients and their families at the end of their life, including management of symptoms, practical issues of law and certification, and effective communication and team working.
      Many people die from consequences of high blood sugar, although more so in low- or middle-income countries compared to the UK. More likely in Joe's case is dying of cardiovascular disease as diabetes increases the risk of heart disease and stroke. Other dangers include limb amputation, blindness, kidney failure and so on.
      The overall risk of dying among people with diabetes is at least double the risk of their peers without diabetes. Despite this, it is only relatively recently that the

palliative care of patients with chronic diseases such as diabetes and COPD (see the case study running through this book) has been emphasised – too often people associate palliative care only with cancer diagnoses and don't consider patients with progressive chronic diseases under this umbrella.

The key message is to remember that diabetes and COPD are progressive conditions, where most patients require intensified therapy over time to control symptoms. Therefore, all team members involved with patients should reflect regularly on their case in order to identify those who may be entering the terminal phase of their condition. If this stage is reached, consideration then needs to be given to how best to share this information with the patient and his/her family. Only if this happens can it be ensured that patients receive high quality, planned palliative care.

Case study: MRSA

Anita Khan, 26 years old, was admitted with acute appendicitis. She was previously fit and healthy. She underwent an emergency appendicectomy and was recovering well at home. However, Anita started to feel unwell with a fever. She went to her GP and was noted to have developed a wound infection so the practice nurse took a wound swab. The lab results from this swab indicated MRSA. Fortunately, Anita's infection was sensitive to trimethoprim so she was able to be treated at home with oral antibiotics (200 mg bd for 10 days). Her screening swab taken on admission was noted to have been negative.

Anita's wound healed well following treatment with antibiotics and she made an otherwise uneventful recovery.

Approximately 25 to 30 per cent of the general population is thought to be colonised with MRSA bacteria at any given time. Infection with MRSA occurs when the bacteria causes disease in that person. In this case, it is likely that Anita has a hospital-acquired infection. It is estimated that at least 5 per cent of patients undergoing operative intervention will develop a wound infection.

In this case, the impact on this individual has been relatively minimal and short term. This is not the case for all patients that are infected with MRSA. Anita's case is a good example of how hospital-acquired infection needs to be managed at a bigger picture level. It is estimated that every case of MRSA costs the NHS thousands of pounds on top of caring for the patient's original condition (in terms of, for example, extra bed days). Simply accepting that infections happen and treating individual patients is therefore not an acceptable solution. Simply treating Anita's infection is not enough – it will obviously 'treat' her but it will not contribute to decreasing the infection rate for subsequent patients.

It may be helpful to consider the management of this problem as an increasing set of concentric circles (Figure 9.1).

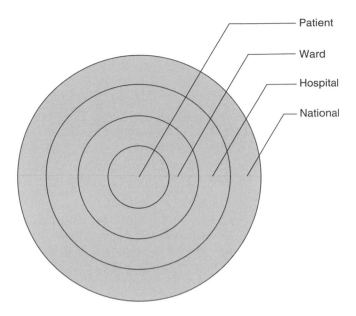

Patient

Ward

Hospital

National

Figure 9.1 Levels of management.

1. Individual patient – Anita's infection needs to be treated with oral or IV antibiotics. Carriers should also be treated with anti-bacterial washes.

2. Ward level – Ward staff need to follow protocols for screening and management of patients, e.g. ensure that appropriate patients are isolated or not admitted unless screening result is available (obviously not possible on emergency admission).

3. Hospital level – New staff induction should include training in infection control procedures. There should be hand dispenser units installed outside wards and hand washing posters to remind staff and visitors of the importance of this. Most hospitals will have a senior nurse who is appointed as an infection control nurse.

4. National and SHA/Health Board NHS level – Hospital infection rates are monitored and hospitals are held accountable not only by the NHS but increasingly by the media and the public. Depending on arrangements, cleaning services may be commissioned. It is also important that information is cascaded to a local level.

This case highlights several key factors that doctors need to be aware of including how the NHS is organised, clinical governance and patient safety. We shall discuss each of these in turn.

How the NHS is organised

In previous chapters we have shown that it is important to take a broader perspective on health than that of the medical model. This leads to viewing the individual as a whole person and thus tackling an illness or problem in three ways: physical, psychological and environmental/social. The extent to which each of these three will be addressed depends on several factors, including where the patient presents. To help put this into context, it is helpful to know a little about how UK healthcare is organised.

A post-war ideal in the UK was that good healthcare should be available to all regardless of wealth. Thus, on 5 July 1948, the then health secretary, Aneurin Bevan, officially founded the National Health Service (NHS). For the first time hospitals, doctors, nurses, pharmacists, opticians and dentists were brought together under one umbrella organisation that was free for all to access at the point of delivery. The service is financed by the state through taxation. Healthcare policy varies slightly throughout the UK, as Scotland and Wales have devolved parliaments.

The Department of Health sets overall policy on all health issues, including public health matters and the health consequences of environmental and food issues. It is also responsible for the provision of health services, a function which it discharges through the National Health Service (NHS) including independent contractors such as General Medical Practitioners (GPs), dentists, pharmacists and opticians. The Department of Health (DoH: **www.dh.gov.uk**) and the other UK health departments – remember healthcare delivery varies by UK country (England, Scotland, Wales and Northern Ireland) – provide guidance for providing high-quality patient care (e.g. healthcare professional training, clinical standards, evidence-based guidelines).

The DoH also sets out schemes rewarding healthcare deliverers for how well they care for patients. One such scheme is the Quality Outcomes Framework (QOF), aimed at general practices (GPs) (see also Chapter 5 and **www.nice.org.uk/aboutnice/qof/qof.jsp**). The QOF contains clinical and health improvement indicators, which cover clinical care (e.g. coronary heart disease, heart failure, hypertension), organisational domains (e.g. record keeping, education and training), patient experience and additional services (e.g. maternity services).

The NHS is structured to provide primary, secondary and tertiary care. Primary care is largely provided in the community and is where most illness first presents and, in fact, where most illness is managed. The primary care GP provides a 'gatekeeper' function to the NHS, dealing with illness in the primary care setting where possible and referring patients to secondary or tertiary care when more specialist investigation or treatment is required. Secondary care is generally provided within local hospitals and tertiary care within specialised regional centres. However, it is also worth noting that the barriers between primary, secondary and tertiary care have begun to blur, with, for example, hospital consultants holding clinics in community-based health centres, and GPs developing specialist interests and services in specific areas such as heart disease.

Approximately 90 per cent of doctor–patient consultations in the UK occur within the primary care setting. A report of the monthly prevalence estimates of illness presentation indicated that, for every 1000 adults, 750 report symptoms, 250 consulted a primary care doctor one or more times per month, nine were admitted to hospital, five were referred onto another doctor, and one was referred to a university medical centre. Compare these figures, published in 1961 (White *et al.*, 1961), with a comparative report of US data, published in 2001 (Figure 9.2).

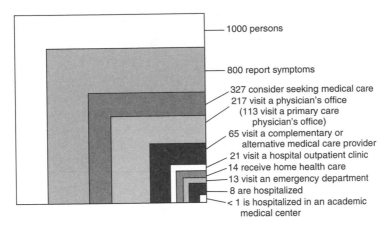

Figure 9.2 Where patients present. Results of a reanalysis of the monthly prevalence of illness in the community and the roles of various sources of healthcare.

Source: Green *et al.*, 2001. Reproduced with permission.

Although the 2001 (Green *et al.*, 2001) figures include children as well as adults, the estimated proportions of persons reporting symptoms, visiting a doctor, receiving care in a hospital and receiving care in an academic medical centre have changed little in 40 years. The authors suggest that this lack of change may represent stability of these proportions, perhaps because the interactions between people and the healthcare system are driven by preferences and needs that persist despite changes in the organisation of healthcare. However, it may be that developments in the healthcare system have had offsetting effects. For example, an increase in the proportion of older persons with chronic diseases may have resulted in more office visits and hospital stays, but cost containment by hospitals and the shifting of care back to the community may have moderated these effects.

Effective delivery of healthcare requires input from a large number of professionals and associated staff. For example, GPs, general dental practitioners (GDPs), out-of-hours service (NHS 24/NHS Direct), practice nurses, district nurses, health visitors, midwives, pharmacists, allied health professionals (e.g. physiotherapists, occupational therapists) and administrative staff all work within the primary care setting. Secondary and tertiary care also requires similar teams of healthcare staff in order to deliver the best possible healthcare. Different professional groups within the NHS have their own professional and regulatory bodies which provide guidance on practice (e.g. the General Medical Council, the Nursing and Midwifery Council). Without exception, anyone entering medicine is required to work as part of a much larger, multi-disciplinary team.

Clinical governance

Clinical governance, the framework through which NHS organisations are accountable for continuously improving the quality of their services and safeguarding high standards of care, is discussed in some detail in Chapter 5. Here we relate clinical governance to Case 2. In Anita's case, doctors and hospital managers should be constantly seeking to decrease their incidence of hospital-acquired infection and specifically MRSA. They should be checking that staff adhere to screening protocols, and address this if there is a gap between guidelines and practice. Remember, just because guidance and policies exist does not mean that people are following them!

With regards to your own clinical practice you should develop an attitude whereby you are continually striving to improve the quality of care that you deliver and regularly reflect on your own practice. This can be done in a variety of ways.

- *Clinical audit* – formally comparing your care to recognised best practice. See Chapter 5 for more discussion of clinical audit.

- *Significant event analysis* (SEA) – an educational tool which can be used by a team to encourage reflection and aid understanding when things go wrong. It can also be used to reflect on those things that go well. Significant event analysis, also referred to as significant event audit, typically has seven stages: awareness and prioritisation of a significant event, information gathering, a facilitated team-based meeting, analysis of the significant event, agree, implement and monitor change, write it up, report, share and review.

- *Appraisal and revalidation* – Appraisal is a developmental and supportive process where a doctor can reflect on their performance with one of their own peer group. Appraisal is well established as a tool for professional development in primary care and is now also universal in the hospital setting. An 'enhanced', more robust version of appraisal is likely to be a cornerstone of the revalidation process for all doctors (i.e. it is proposed that all doctors will need to undergo the more robust process of revalidation in order that they may continue to hold their licence to practice as a doctor). Some doctors are concerned that a less reflective and more challenging version of appraisal blurs the dividing line with assessment – at the time of writing this book the debate continues.

- *Patient satisfaction questionnaires* – These are one form of outcome measurement, used to measure how satisfied patients are with their visit to the doctor. They are ideal to capture feedback from patients who have experienced your services and are in a position to reflect on their satisfaction with the care they received. Patient satisfaction questionnaires tend to measure factors such as the doctor–patient relationship, the communication skills (e.g. listening) and empathy of the doctor, but may also include questions on the service received (e.g. time to wait, how long it took to get an appointment).

Patient safety

Last, but by no means least, we should touch on the concept of patient safety. In the case we highlighted above, the patient came to harm as a result of her hospital admission. Healthcare is a high hazard industry: it is estimated that at least 10 per cent of patient contacts result in harm to patients and of those, at least half should be preventable. However, many patient safety incidents go unrecognised, hence the need for systems such as the Yellow Card Scheme to report medicine side-effects (**http://yellowcard.mhra.gov.uk/the-yellow-card-scheme**) and initiatives such as the National Patient Safety Alliance (**www.npsa.nhs.uk**). These examples demonstrate how the NHS is attempting to move to a culture where people share their mistakes so that we can learn from them (and hopefully not repeat them).

You may be studying medicine at a university which has adopted the WHO Patient Safety Curriculum Guide for Medical Schools, published in 2009 (**www.who. int/patientsafety/education/curriculum/en/index.html**) (WHO, 2009b), which aims to encourage and facilitate the teaching of patient safety topics to medical students. Whether or not you are receiving this precise curriculum, you will most certainly be learning about patient safety as this is everywhere in clinical medicine. Good medical practice encompasses all the principles of patient safety. However, on the wards, in theatre or in the general practice surgery, those principles are often tacit or unspoken.

As a medical student or junior doctor, you have a responsibility not to undertake tasks for which you are not adequately trained. In previous years, there may have been a culture of 'see one, do one, teach one' but now doctors would only be expected to do things for which they are competent and trained. Tragic patient safety errors, like that of Wayne Jowett, a teenager who died after doctors injected a powerful cancer treatment drug into his spine instead of a vein (to find out more use 'Wayne Jowett' as a search term) would hopefully not happen now but do demonstrate the 'Swiss cheese' model of patient safety (Reason, 2000). According to this metaphor, in a complex system, hazards are prevented from causing human harm by a series of barriers. Each barrier has unintended weaknesses, or holes – hence the similarity with Swiss cheese. These weaknesses are inconstant – i.e. the holes open and close at random. When by chance all holes are aligned, the hazard reaches the patient and causes harm. This model draws attention to the healthcare system, as opposed to the individual, and to randomness, as opposed to deliberate action, in the occurrence of medical errors. To bring this back to the Wayne Jowett case, in attempting to prevent re-occurrence many changes had to be made not only to individual hospital systems but also to medical equipment used nationally. Search the internet to find a diagram of James Reason's 'Swiss cheese' model.

And finally . . .

The final thing we wanted to include was some collective 'top tips' for medical students progressing onto Foundation Years training (and later . . .). These are based on our own experiences of working as doctors and are things we either realised along the way or wish someone had told us sooner!

- Always be looking forward – think about what you need to do to take the next step in your career, for example if you need to try and get a publication, is there someone looking for help with writing? Look for opportunities to do research, even as a student. For example, some medical schools offer studentships in clinical medicine and medical education. These are an excellent opportunity to gain experience of research/audit, and often lead to conference presentations and publications.

- Work–life balance – first, be realistic in what you have to and want to do and the time you have to do it. Second, don't neglect your leisure time and your personal life – these are the things that keep you sane and make life worth living. If you don't believe us, go and read up about burnout in the medical profession.

- If you're not well enough to work, call in sick. If you are not fit to be working, then you have a responsibility not to be at work. Sometimes in medicine we have a belief that if we are not at work then the world will end. It does not. You do not want to make a mistake and possibly cause a patient harm because you are feeling unwell. Seek proper help (i.e. don't just phone a friend, make an appointment with your GP) if you are really unwell – you will not get a prize for soldiering on, contaminating your colleagues and patients with some unpleasant virus or feeling worse and worse about your own competence by only barely managing to function.

- Work as part of a team – it's a cliché, but there is no 'I' in 'TEAM'. And make sure you 'befriend' the nurses. Why? Other than simply out of professional respect, you will find that nurses are often based on wards for a lot longer than junior doctors on rotations. Experienced nurses are often a great source of local information and support for you. As a newly qualified doctor one of the biggest mistakes you can make is to play the 'but I am the doctor' card. Try it once, and you will see what we mean.

- If you don't know, ask for help – better than making a big mistake that could harm a patient and wreck your career. Know when to ask for help – recognise the limits of your own competence – and who to ask. Do not be afraid to say to a patient 'I don't know, I'll need to discuss this with a colleague/look up guidance'.

- Learn from the advice you are given so you don't keep asking the same question(s).

- Treat people as you would want you or your family treated – that applies to colleagues and patients. Basically, treat patients as people not as collections of symptoms.

- Don't be afraid to think outside the box – just because that's the way everyone else has done things doesn't necessarily mean it's the best or only way to do things (though sometimes it is).

- Question if you think something is wrong – just use your highly developed communication skills to do it. But seriously, if you think something isn't right then you have a duty as a doctor to raise your concerns. And if you're ever not sure what's the right thing to do then speak to your defence union – that's what you pay them for!

References

Ajzen, I (1985) From intentions to actions: a theory of planned behavior, in Kuhl, J and Beckmann, J (eds) *Action Control: From Cognition to Behavior*. New York: Springer-Verlag. For more information see: www.people.umass.edu/aizen/faq.html

Alemayehu, B and Warner, KE (2004) The lifetime distribution of health care costs. *Health Services Research*, 39: 627–642.

Andermann, A, Blancquaert, I, Beauchamp, S and Déry, V (2008) Revisiting Wilson and Jungner in the genomic age: a review of screening criteria over the past 40 years. *Bulletin of the World Health Organization*, 86(4): 241–320. www.who.int/bulletin/volumes/86/4/07-050112/en

Bandura, A (1977) Self-efficacy: toward a unifying theory of behavioral change. *Psychological Review*, 84: 191–215. For more information see: www.des.emory.edu/mfp/self-efficacy.html

Baum, M (1986) Do we need informed consent? *The Lancet*, 2(8512): 911–912.

Becker, MH (1974) The health belief model and personal health behavior. *Health Education Monographs*, 2: 324–473.

Blaxter, M (1990) *Health and Lifestyles*. London: Tavistock Routledge.

Boddington, P and Podpadec, T (1999) Measuring quality of life in theory and in practice, in Kuhse, H and Singer, P (eds) *Bioethics: An Anthology* (Oxford: Blackwell), pp 273–282.

Bourdieu, P (1986) The forms of capital, in Richardson, JG (ed) *Handbook for Theory and Research for the Sociology of Education*. New York: Greenwood.

Bunn, F, Collier, T, Frost, C, Ker, K, Roberts, I and Wentz, R (2003) Traffic calming for the prevention of road traffic injuries: systematic review and meta-analysis. *Injury Prevention*, 9(3): 200–204.

Burney, P and Jarvis, D (2006) The burden of COPD in the UK. *National Knowledge Week of COPD 13–17 Nov 2006*. www.library.nhs.uk/respiratory/ViewResource.aspx?resID=187247

Burr, ML, Wat, D, Evans, C, Dunstan, FDJ and Doull, IJM (2006) Asthma prevalence in 1973, 1988 and 2003. *Thorax*, April, 61(4): 296–299.

Butler, RN (1987) Ageism, in Maddox, GL and Atchley, RC (eds) *The Encyclopedia of Aging*. New York: Springer.

Cappuccio, FP (2004) Epidemiologic transition, migration and cardiovascular disease. *International Journal of Epidemiology*, 33: 387–388.

Chen, LS and Kaphingst, KA (2010) Risk perceptions and family history of lung cancer: difference by smoking status. *Public Health Genomics*, 14(1): 26–34.

Cooper, C (1999) *Continuing Care of Sick Children: Examining the Impact of Chronic Illness*. Chichester: Wiley.

Covey, SR (2004) *The 7 Habits of Highly Effective People*. New York: Simon & Schuster (15th Anniversary Edition).

Craig, JV and Smyth, RL (eds) (2002) *The Evidence-based Practice Manual for Nurses*. Edinburgh: Churchill Livingstone.

Dahlgren, G and Whitehead, M (1991) *Policies and Strategies to Promote Social Equity in Health*. Stockholm: Stockholm Institute for Future Studies.

de la Jara, R (2007) IQ Comparison Site, www.iqcomparisonsite.com

Department of Health Expert Group (2000) An organisation with a memory. *The Stationery Office Limited*, www.dh.gov.uk/en/Publicationsandstatistics/Publications/PublicationsPolicyAndGuidance/DH_4065083.

Downie, RS, Fyfe, C and Tannahill, A (1990) *Health Promotion: Models and Values*. Oxford: Oxford University Press.

Dunn-Geier, BJ, McGrath, PJ, Rourke, BP, Latter, J and D'Astous, J (1986) Adolescent chronic pain: the ability to cope. *Pain*, 26(1): 23–32.

EMIS (2011) *Immunisation Schedule (UK)*. Egton Medical Information Systems Limited. www.patient.co.uk/doctor/Immunisation-Schedule-(UK).htm

Ferguson, E, James, D, O'Hehir, F and Sanders, A (2003) Pilot study of the roles of personality, references, and personal statements in relation to performance over the five years of a medical degree. *British Medical Journal*, 326: 429–432.

Fries, JF (1980) Aging, natural death, and the compression of morbidity. *N Engl J Med*, 303: 130–135.

Gibbs, G (1988) *Learning by Doing: A Guide to Teaching and Learning Methods*. Further Education Unit, Oxford Polytechnic: Oxford.

GMC (2006) *Good Medical Practice* (GMC), www.gmc-uk.org/guidance/good_medical_practice.asp

GMC (2009) *Tomorrow's Doctors*, www.gmc-uk.org/static/documents/content/TomorrowsDoctors_2009.pdf

GMC/MSC (2009) *Medical Students: Professional Values and Fitness to Practise*, www.gmc-uk.org/static/documents/content/GMC_Medical_Students.pdf

Green, LA, Fryer, GE, Yawn, BP and Lanier, D (2001) The ecology of medical care revisited. *New England Journal of Medicine*, 344: 2021–2025.

Greenwood, E (1957) Attributes of a profession. *Social Work*, 2(3): 45–55.

Guyatt, GH, Sackett, DL and Cook, DJ (1993a) Users' guide to the medical literature. II. How to use an article about therapy or prevention. A. Are the results of the study valid? *JAMA*, 270: 2589–2601.

Guyatt, GH, Sackett, DL and Cook, DJ (1993b) Users' guide to the medical literature. II. How to use an article about therapy or prevention. B. What were the results and will they help me in caring for my patients? *JAMA*, 271: 59–63.

Hales, CN and Barker, DJ (1992) Type 2 (non-insulin-dependent) diabetes mellitus: the thrifty phenotype hypothesis. *Diabetologia*, 35 (7): 595–601.

Hawthorne, K, Rahman, J and Pill, R (2003) Working with Bangladeshi patients in Britain: perspectives from primary care. *Family Practice*, 20: 185–191.

Helman, C (2007) *Culture, Health and Illness*, 5th edition. London: Hodder Arnold.

HMG (2000) *Adults with Incapacity (Scotland) Act*. Stationary Office.

HMSO (1956) *Clean Air Legislation*, www.legislation.gov.uk/ukpga/1956/52/pdfs/ukpga_19560052_en.pdf

Holmes, TH and Rahe, RH (1967) The social readjustment rating scale. *Journal of Psychosomatic Research*, 11(2): 213–218.

Johnston, M, Pollard, B, Morrison, V and MacWalter, R (2005) Functional limitations and survival following stroke: psychological and clinical predictors of 3-year outcome. *International Journal of Behavioral Medicine*, 11: 187–196.

Juniper, EF, Guyatt, GH, Epstein, RS, Ferrie, PJ, Jaeschke, R and Hiller, TK (1992) Evaluation of impairment of health-related quality of life in asthma: development of a questionnaire for use in clinical trials. *Thorax*, 47: 76–83.

Killeen, D (1994) Food and nutrition, in Fyfe, G (ed) *Poor and Paying for it: The Price of Living on a Low Income*. Glasgow: Scottish Consumer Council.

Klegon, D (1978) The sociology of the professions, an emerging perspective. *Work and Occupations*, August, 5(3): 259–283.

Kübler-Ross, E (1973) *On Death and Dying*. New York: Routledge.

Lazarus, RS and Folkman, S (1984) *Stress, Appraisal and Coping*. New York: Springer.

Leventhal, H, Diefenback, M and Leventhal, E (1992) Illness cognition: using common sense to understand treatment adherence and affect cognition interactions. *Cognitive Therapy & Research*, 16(2): 143–163.

Lingard, L, Espin, S, Whyte, S, Regehr, G, Baker, GR, Reznick, R *et al.* (2004) Communication failures in the operating room: an observational classification of recurrent types and effects. *Qual Saf Health Care*, 13: 330–334.

Lubitz, JG and Riley, GF (1993) Trends in Medicare payments in the last year of life. *New England Journal of Medicine*, 328: 1092–1096.

Macdonald, KM (1995) *The Sociology of the Professions*. London: Sage.

Macintyre, S, Ellaway, A, Der, G, Ford, G and Hunt, K (1998) Do housing tenure and car access predict health because they are simply markers of income or self-esteem? A Scottish study. *Journal of Epidemiology and Community Health*, 52: 657–664.

Mackenbach, JP, Stirbu, I, Roskam, AR, Schaap, MM, Menvielle, G, Leinsalu, M and others (2008) Socioeconomic inequalities in health in 22 European countries. *New England Journal of Medicine*, 358: 2468–2481.

Mahoney, FI and Barthel, DW (1965) Functional evaluation: the Barthel Index. *Maryland State Medical Journal*, February, 14: 61–65.

Marmot, MG, Rose, G, Shipley, M and Hamilton, PJ (1978) Employment grade and coronary heart disease in British civil servants. *Journal of Epidemiology and Community Health*, 32(4): 244–249.

McKinstrey, B (1992) Paternalism and the doctor–patient relationship in general practice. *British Journal of General Practice*, 42: 340–342.

Mechanic, D (1968) *Medical Sociology*. London: Free Press.

Mikhail, GW (2005) Coronary heart disease in women. *BMJ*, 331: 467–468.

Moynihan, R (2003) The making of a disease: female sexual dysfunction. *BMJ*, 326: 45–47.

Naidoo, J and Wills, J (2005). *Public Health and Health Promotion: Developing Practice*, 2nd edition. Bailliere-Tindale.

National Statistics Online (2010), www.statistics.gov.uk/cci/nugget.asp?id=949

Newman, S, Steed, L and Mulligan, K (2004) Self-management interventions for chronic illness. *The Lancet*, 364, 1523–1537.

NHS Quality Improvement Scotland (NHS QIS), www.healthcareimprovementscotland.org/home.aspx

Offer, D and Sabshin, M (eds) (1991) *The Diversity of Normal Behaviour*. New York: Basic Books.

Ogden, J (2007) *Health Psychology: A Textbook*. Buckingham: Oxford University Press.

Ottawa Charter for Health Promotion (1986) *First International Conference on Health Promotion*. Ottawa Charter for Health Promotion, www.who.int/hpr/NPH/docs/ottawa_charter_hp.pdf

Paling, J (2003) Strategies to help patients understand risks. *BMJ*, 327: 745–748.

Parsons, T (1975) The sick role and the role of the physician reconsidered. *Health and Society*, 53(3): 257–278.

Prochaska, J and DiClemente, C (1984) *The Transtheoretical Approach: Crossing Traditional Boundaries of Therapy*. Homewood IL: Dow Jones-Irwin. For more information, see www.uri.edu/research/cprc/transtheoretical.htm

Reason, J (2000) Human error: models and management. *BMJ,* 320: 768–770.

Rickard, K (1988) The occurrence of maladaptive health-related behaviours and teacher-rated conduct problems in children of chronic low back pain patients. *Journal of Behavioral Medicine*, 11: 107–116.

Salmon, P (2000) *Psychology of Medicine and Surgery: A Guide for Psychologists, Counsellors, Nurses and Doctors*. Chichester: John Wiley and Sons.

Schön, D (1983) *The Reflective Practitioner*. Basic Books: New York.

Schwartz, GE (1982) Testing the biopsychosocial model: the ultimate challenge facing behavioral medicine? *Journal of Consulting and Clinical Psychology*, 50: 1040–1053.

Schwarzer, R and Jerusalem, M (1995) Generalized Self-Efficacy Scale, in Weinman, J, Wright, S and Johnston, M (eds) *Measures in Health Psychology: A User's Portfolio. Causal and Control Beliefs*. Windsor: NFER-Nelson.

Scottish Deans' Medical Curriculum Group (various) *The Scottish Doctor Project*. Scottish Deans' Medical Curriculum Group, www.scottishdoctor.org

Senior, P and Bhopal, R (1994) Ethnicity as a variable in epidemiological research. *British Medical Journal*, 309, 327–330.

Shah, P and Mountain, D (2007) The medical model is dead – long live the medical model. *British Journal of Psychiatry*, 191: 375–377.

Shults, R, Elder, R, Sleet, D *et al*. (2001) Reviews of evidence regarding interventions to reduce alcohol-impaired driving. *American Journal of Preventive Medicine*, 21(4 Suppl): 66–88.

Skinner, EA, Edge, K, Altman, J and Sherwood, H (2003) Searching for the structure of coping: a review and critique of category systems for classifying ways of coping. *Psychological Bulletin*, 129: 216–269.

Steinberg, L (2007) *Adolescence*. New York: McGraw-Hill.

Szasz, TS and Hollander, MH (1956) A contribution to the philosophy of medicine: the basic models of the doctor–patient relationship. *Archives of Internal Medicine,* 97: 585–592.

Tallis, R (2004) *Hippocratic Oaths: Medicine and its Discontents*. Tunbridge Wells: Atlantic Books.

Taylor, RJ, Smith, BH and van Teijlingen, ER (eds) (2003) *Health and Illness in the Community*. Oxford: Oxford University Press.

Townsend, P and Davidson, N (eds) (1982) *Inequalities in Health: The Black Report*. Penguin: Harmondsworth.

Tudor Hart, J (1971) The inverse care law. *The Lancet*, 27 February 1971.

UK Government, *What is Stress?* Health & Safety Executive, www.hse.gov.uk/stress/ furtheradvice/whatisstress.htm

UKGov Mental Capacity Act (England and Wales) (2005). HMSO, www.legislation.gov.uk/ukpga/2005/9/contents

van Teijlingen, E, Lowis, G, McCaffery, P and Porter, M (eds) (2004) *Midwifery and the Medicalization of Childbirth: Comparative Perspectives*. Hauppauge NY: Nova Science Publishers.

Waddell, G and Burton, AK (2006) *Is Work Good for Your Health and Well-Being?* London: The Stationery Office, www.dwp.gov.uk/docs/hwwb-is-work-good-for-you.pdf

Wakefield, AJ, Murch, SH, Anthony, A and others (1998) Ileal-lymphoid-nodular hyperplasia, non-specific colitis, and pervasive developmental disorder in children. *Lancet*, 351 (9103): 637–641.

Ware, JE and Sherbourne, CD (1992) The MOS 36-item Short-Form health survey (SF-36): I. Conceptual framework and item selection. *Medical Care*, 30, 473–483.

Weinstein, ND (1987) Unrealistic optimism about susceptibility to health problems: conclusions from a community-wide sample. *Journal of Behavioral Medicine*, 10: 481–490.

White, KL, Williams, TF and Greenberg, BG (1961). The ecology of medical care. *New England Journal of Medicine*, 265: 885–892.

Wilkinson, R and Marmot, M (eds) (2003) *Social Determinants of Health: The Solid Facts.* Copenhagen: World Health Organization.

Wilson, JMG and Jungner, G (1968) *Principles and Practice of Screening for Disease.* Geneva: WHO. Available from: http://whqlibdoc.who.int/php/WHO_PHP_34.pdf

World Health Organization (1948) *Constitution of the World Health Organization.* Geneva: WHO (as adopted by the International Health Conference, New York, 19–22 June 1946; signed 22 July 1946 by the representatives of 61 states (Official Records of the World Health Organization, no. 2, p. 100) and entered into force 7 April 1948), www.who.int/rarebooks/official_records/constitution.pdf

World Health Organization (2002) *WHO Gender Policy: Integrating Gender Perspectives in the Work of WHO*. World Health Organization, www.who.int/gender/documents/engpolicy.pdf

World Health Organization (2006) *Commission on Social Determinants of Health: Final Report*. Geneva: World Health Organization, www.who.int/social_determinants/thecommission/finalreport/en/index.html

World Health Organization (2007) *Composition of World Health Expenditures: Government Spend on Healthcare*. Geneva: WHO, www.who.int/nha/en

World Health Organization (2007) *Total Expenditure on Health per Capita. Government Spend on Healthcare*. Geneva: WHO, www.who.int/nha/en

World Health Organization (2008a) *The Global Burden of Disease: 2004 Update.*

Geneva: WHO, www.who.int/healthinfo/global_burden_disease/GBD_report_2004update_full.pdf

World Health Organization (2008b) *Closing the Gap in a Generation: Health Equity through Action on the Social Determinants of Health*. Geneva: WHO.

World Health Organization (2009a) *Global Health Risks: Mortality and Burden of Disease Attributable to Selected Major Risks*. Geneva: WHO.

World Health Organization (2009b) *Patient Safety Curriculum Guide for Medical Schools*, www.who.int/patientsafety/education/curriculum/en/index.html

Young, ME, Norman, GR and Humphreys, KR (2008) The role of medical language in changing public perceptions of illness. *PLoS ONE*, 3(12): e3875.

Zigmond, AS and Snaith, RP (1983) The hospital anxiety and depression scale. *Acta Psychiatrica Scandinavica*, 67: 361–370.

Zola, IK (1973) Pathways from the doctor: From person to patient. *Social Science & Medicine*, 7: 677–689.

Index

activities of daily living (ADL) 149, 150
adaptation 40, 57
addictions 72
adolescence 31–2
adulthood: early 32–4; middle 34
Adults with Incapacity (Scotland) Act
    (2000) 163
adverse incidents 135–6
age: health and 13, 17–18, 70; old 34–6;
    see also children; elderly patients
ageism 34
air pollution 16, 17
alcoholism 47
Alzheimer's disease 26, 36
amyotrophic lateral sclerosis (ALS) 85
ante-natal screening 154
antibiotics 10
anxiety 30, 37, 39, 56, 58, 105, 146, 151
appraisal 174
assisted suicide 154
asthma 32, 53, 55, 62, 84, 107, 128
Asthma Quality of Life Questionnaire 151
attachment 29
attention 26
attitudes towards health and illness 13–14, 41
avian flu 99, 111

babies *see* infants
bad news, breaking 10
Barthel Index of Activities of Daily Living 150
behaviour change, models of 48–52
behavioural risk factors 46–7
bereavement 33, 35–6, 40
Bevan, Aneurin 172
Bhopal disaster 114
Big Five personality dimensions 38
biopsychosocial model 11–12, 15, 26, 35, 45
birth 28–31

Black Report 87
blame culture 65
blood-borne viruses (BBV) 16
body mass index (BMI) 88
borderline personality disorder 47
Bowlby, John 28, 29
breaking bad news 10
breast cancer screening 104
British National Formulary (BNF) 94, 159
Broad Street pump cholera outbreak 17

Call and Recall System 104, 105
cancer, childhood 30
cardiovascular disease 30, 88; diabetes
    and 169; ethnic group 68, 69; gender
    and 71; risk factors 46; stress and 54
case-control study 127, 128
Chernobyl nuclear disaster 17–18, 113,
    114–15
children: cancer 30; chronic illness and
    psychosocial disturbance 30; early 28–31;
    key developmental stages 28–9; obesity
    in 88; routine immunisation schedule 102
cholera 17
chronic fatigue syndrome 76
chronic obstructive pulmonary disease
    (COPD) 13, 16, 46, 48, 124; activity
    limitation 147–8; birth weight and 30;
    case study 23, 42, 59, 97, 117, 138–9,
    145, 157; clinical effectiveness and 90;
    epidemiology 85–6; evidence-based
    guidelines 97; management 138–9;
    palliative care 170; rehabilitation 168;
    self-management programmes 58; sick
    role 76; tertiary prevention 106
Clean Air legislation (1956) (UK) 17
Cleanliness Champions 108
clinical audit 93–4, 134–5, 174

clinical audit cycle 93
clinical effectiveness 89, 96; importance of 90–1; quality improvement activities 91–2
clinical governance 173–4
clinical guidelines 89, 92–3, 132
clinical research and ethics 132–4
Clostridium difficile infections 110, 111
Cochrane Collaboration 132
Cochrane Library 59, 132
Cochrane Reviews 132
cognitive development 28
cognitive psychology 26
cohort study 127–8
communicable diseases: notification 108; preventive measures 109
communication 159; disability and 156; doctor–patient 73–4; ethnicity and barriers to 69; inter-professional 72, 168; non-verbal 73; outcome measures and 55; patient safety and 168–9; with children 31
community 66
community-based diabetes nurse specialist 168
competition between professions 63–4
compression of morbidity 151–2
content analysis 128
contraception, female 20, 128
coping 40, 52, 57; stress and 36–7; strategies 31, 37, 57–8
cost-benefit analysis 96
cost effectiveness analysis 96
cost-minimisation analysis 96
cost-utility analysis 96
critical appraisal 129–30
Critical Appraisal Skills Programme 130
crystallised intelligence 34
cultural competency 69–70
cultural norms 8–9
culture 65

deafness 146
death, causes, global 81–2
degenerative diseases 11
deliberate self-harm (DSH) 47
delusions 27

demand 95–97
denial 39
Department of Health 172
dependency ratio 70
depression 33, 36, 37, 38, 39, 47, 146, 149, 151; in chronic illness 56; in women 71
developmental delay 29–30
developmental milestones 29
developmental psychology 27
developmental window hypothesis 30
diabetes clinic 51, 168, 169
diabetes rehabilitation team 168
Diabetes UK 169
diabetes, type II 13, 30, 31, 32, 34, 46, 73, 88, 107; case study 160, 161–70
disability 142–4; assessment of 149–50; intervention in 156; models of 76–7, 144–9; preventing 153–5; severe 155
Disability Discrimination Act (1995) 142, 145
disabling illnesses 11
disease control 108
disease elimination 108
disease mongering 15
disease prevention 100, 101–7
disease surveillance 84
divided attention 26
divorce 33
doctor–patient relationship 10, 54, 73, 107, 160, 162, 167, 174
double-blind randomised controlled trials 125–6
Down's syndrome 154
drinking water 114
drug culture 65

education: adjustment to birth of baby and 33; differences in 68, disability and 144; ethnicity and 65; health and 20; psycho-education 58; *see also* health education
elderly patients, 'normal' health of 13
environmental disasters 17–18
environmental hazards 14–15, 16, 18, 113–16
environmental illness, recognition of 116
environmental influences on health 15–18
epidemic curve 110, 111
epidemiology 84–6

Equality Act (2010) 142–3, 145, 148
Erikson, Erik 28
ethnicity 66, 67; health and 68–70; language
  and 67, 68, 69, 74
ethnography 128
etiquette 155–6
eugenics 145
evidence: hard-copy 123–4; internet 122–3;
  sources of 122–4
evidence-based medicine 10, 11, 76, 89, 90, 92
expected loss 40
expert patient self-management
  programme 58–9
exposure 113–15
exposure control 115–16
exposure pathways 114–15

family planning 20
feminism 63
fight or flight response 54
fitness to work 176
five stages of grief 35–6, 57
fluid intelligence 34
focus groups 128
Fukushima nuclear disaster 18
functional capacity 150
Functional Motor Test 150
functionalism 63

gender 12; influence on health 12–13, 70–1
General Medical Council 173
General Medical Services Contract 92
General Self-Efficacy Scale (GSE) 50
Gibbs' reflective cycle 137–8
glaucoma screening 104
Good Medical Practice 142
grief: atypical 26; stages of 35–6, 57
guidance-cooperation model 10

hallucinations 27, 73
harm, definition 16
hazards: biological 16; definition 15;
  environmental 14–15, 16, 18, 113–16;
  healthcare 175; occupational 113, 115;
  perception of 16; recognition of 115
health: global patterns 81–3; influences
on 86–9; WHO definition of 21–2, 26,
  81, 88
health and safety 16
Health Belief Model 48
health economics 95–6
health education 101, 112–13
health gradient 68
health needs assessment 95, 96–7
health promotion 34, 74, 100–1
health protection 100–1, 107
health risks 82
healthcare: decision-making 94–5;
  equality 90; expenditure 18–20, 94;
  global patterns of 81–3; inequality 90;
  system effectiveness 19; UK, organisation
  of 22–3
health-related behaviour 45–7; factors
  influencing 47–8; models of 48–52
health-related QoL (HRQoL) 150–1
health-seeking behaviour 13–14
heart rate, normal 8
Hepatitis B (HBV) 16
Hepatitis C (HCV) 16
Herriot, Kenny 13
hierarchies of evidence 131–2
high culture 65
HIV infection 16, 76, 82, 83, 108, 146
homeostasis 13, 33
homosexuality 8–9
Hospital Anxiety & Depression Scale 56
human immunodeficiency virus (HIV) see HIV
  infection
'humors' (Greek) 10

Ideas, Concerns and Expectations (ICE) 162–3
illness behaviour 41
illness vs disease 74–7
immunisation 101–3, 109
immunisation schedule, routine childhood 102
impairments 143
IMRaD convention 129
in-depth interviews 128
incidence 84–5
individual influences on health 12–15
infants: adjustment to having 33;
  low-birth-weight 13; mortality rates 18

infectious diseases 82; control of 108
informed consent 125, 134
intention-behaviour gap 49
International Classification of Functions (ICF) Framework 147–8
internet as source of evidence 122–3
inverse care law 68
IQ distribution 8
irritable bowel syndrome 53, 162

journals 168; as source of evidence 123–4
Jowett, Wayne 175
Jung, Carl 38

Kayan tribe, Thailand 9

labelling, negative 145
labour pain 74
language 27; culture and 65; ethnicity and 67, 68, 69, 74
lay risk perceptions 14, 15
learning 27
Life Events Scale 39
life expectancy 16, 18, 82, 151
life stages 28
Local Research Ethics Committee (LREC) 133–4
London fog 17, 18, 113
loss 40
lung cancer, risk of 14
Lyme disease 108

macro level of study 62, 72–3
marriage 65; psychology of 32–3
Marxism 63
medical history 160–1
medical labelling 15
medical model 9–11, 18, 21, 54, 76, 107, 144–5
medical sociology 71–2
medicalisation 72
medically unexplained symptoms 53
memory 27
Mental Capacity Act 2005 (England and Wales) 163
mental-state examination 163

methicillin-resistance *Staphylococcus aureus* (MRSA) *see* MRSA
micro level of human interaction 62, 73–4
mind-body interactions 45
MMR vaccination 103
model of health 11, 62
morbidity, compression of 151–2
motherhood, adjustment to 33
motor neurone disease (amyotrophic lateral sclerosis; ALS) 85
MRSA 99, 110, 111; case study 160, 170–1, 174
multi-disciplinary pain management programmes 58
MumsNet 67
mutual participation model 10
Myers-Briggs Type Indicator (MBTI) 38

National Childbirth Trust 67
National Health Service 19; organisation of 171–3
National Health Service Quality Improvement Scotland (NHS QIS) 89, 92
National Institute for Health and Clinical Excellence (NICE) 88, 92, 97, 108, 132, 152, 164
National Patient Safety Agency (NPSA) 132, 136
National Patient Safety Alliance 175
National Research Ethics Service (NRES) 132, 133, 135
natural disasters 18
need 95, 96–7
neglect 33
normal, definition 8–11
notification of diseases 108
Nursing and Midwifery Council 173
nutrition 87–8

obesity 30, 48, 88; childhood 88
occupational stress 27
occupational hazards 113, 115
occupational illness 116
occupational influences on health 15–18
Office for Disability Issues 144
online learning 168

osteoporosis 71
Ottawa Charter for Health Promotion 100
outbreak investigation and control 110–11
outcome measures 55

pain, definition 54
parenthood, transition to 33
Parsons, Talcott 75, 76
passive immunisation 103
patient expectations 95
patient safety 174–5
patient satisfaction questionnaires 174
PDSA (Plan, Do, Study, Act) cycles 86, 91
peer pressure 16, 49
peer-reviewed journals 76, 123, 133
perceived control 49
perception 26, 27
performance measurement 135
period prevalence 84
personality 27, 37–8; health and 28;
    interaction with early experience 38–41
personality traits 27
personality types 38
phobias 27
physical abuse 33
physical examination, full 163
Piaget, Jean 28
PICO framework 124
planning health services 94–7
point prevalence 84
political and social influences on health 18–21
population demographics 94
population health 81
post-traumatic stress disorder (PTSD) 30
poverty 68; health risks 82
practice nurse 168
pregnancy, termination of 155
prevalence 84–5; of disability 143
preventive measures 109–10
primary care 172, 173
primary prevention 100, 101–3
primordial prevention 100, 101, 107
problem-based small group learning
    (PBSG) 168
problem-solving skills 40
professions, sociology of 63–4

protective factors 40
protocols 92
psycho-educational interventions and
    support 58–9
psychological impact of disease 56–8
psychological model of disability 146–9
psychology applied to medicine 25–6
psychology, definition 26–8
public health: agencies 82; essential elements
    of 80

qualitative methods 125, 128
qualitative research studies 128
quality-adjusted life year (QALY) 96, 152–3
quality improvement activities 91–2
quality improvement tools 93–4
quality of life (QoL) 21–2, 55, 149, 150–1, 155
Quality Outcomes Framework (QOF) 23, 91,
    92–3, 172
quantitative methods 125

race 67
randomised controlled trials (RCTs) 125–7
Redgrave, Sir Steve 13
reflection-in-action 137
reflection-on-action 137
reflective practice 136–8
relationships, psychology of 32–3
relative risk (RR) 84
relaxation training 58
Research Ethics Committee (REC) 132
research methods 124–5
research synthesis 131–2
resilience, development of 39–40
resource allocation 95–6, 152–3
revalidation 174
rheumatoid arthritis 153
risk perceptions 14, 15, 16
risks, health 82; social differentiation in 68
root cause analysis 91

sanctity of life 154–5
schizophrenia 27, 47
scientific method 124; applying 129–31
Scottish Intercollegiate Guidelines Network
    (SIGN) 132

screening programmes 34, 104–6
screening tests 104–5, 106
secondary care 172, 173
secondary prevention 100, 101, 103–6
selective attention 26
self-care 46, 95, 169–70
self-efficacy 49–50
self-injury 47
self-management 46, 58–9
self-regulatory model 52, 53
self-report 150
semiotics 128
severe acute respiratory syndrome (SARS) 111
sex (gender) 12, 70; influence on health 12–13
sexual abuse 33, 40
sick-role behaviour 46, 75–7
significant event analysis (SEA) 174
significant events 135–6
small group learning 168
smallpox vaccine 10
smoking 16; cessation 36, 51–2, 74; Health Belief Model 48; health education 101; infant birth weight and 30; legislation 107; risk perception 13
Snow, Dr John 17
social capital 67
social class 64; mortality and 20
social development 28
social influences on health and illness 11–12
social institutions 64–5
social model 145–6; of disability 155; of health and illness 9–11, 20–1
Social Readjustment Rating Scale (SRRS) 39
social structure 64–5
socio-economics, unhealthy behaviours and 48
Sociology of Health and Illness 71–2
sociology: definition 61–4; fundamental 64–7; importance to medicine 67–8; of professions 63–4
somatisation 53
spina bifida 153
spirometry 117
Stages of Change model 50, 51
statistical process control 91
stereotyping 89: ageism 34; culture and 65; gender 8

stigma 10, 108, 109, 145
stress 27, 36–7, 39; emotions and health 52–3; employment and 72–3; management 27, 58; response and disease processes 54–5
stressors 36–7, 57
substance misuse 47
sudden loss 40
suicide, assisted 154
superstition 10
supply 95
surveillance 108–9
susceptibility to disease 18
Swiss cheese model of patient safety 175
symptom perception 53–4
syphilis 108
systematic reviews 59, 131–2

team working 168–9, 176
tertiary care 172, 173
tertiary prevention 100, 101, 106–7
textbooks as source of evidence 123
Theory of Planned Behaviour (TPB) 48–9
thinking 27
thought-provoking events 135
thrifty phenotype 107
trait models of personality 38
transmission, modes of 108
Transtheoretical Model 50, 51
triage 122
tuberculosis (TB) 108
Type A personality 38
Type B personality 38

'ugly law', Chicago 145
undernourishment 88
undernutrition 82
unemployment, ethnicity and 67
unrealistic optimism 14
utility-based measures 152

value of life debate 154
variation in clinical practice 90
vocations 63
Vygotsky, Lev 28

water, drinking 114

WHO: definition of health 21–2, 26, 81,
    88; Patient Safety Curriculum Guide
    for Medical Schools 175; Weekly
    Epidemiological Record 109
work stress 72–3
working conditions 68
work–life balance 176

workplace: accidents 16, 114; disability
    and 145; exposure in 114;
    hazards 113, 115
World Health Organization *see* WHO

Yellow Card Scheme 175
youth culture 65